Injection Techniques in Orthopaedic and Sports Medicine

SECOND EDITION

Stephanie Saunders

FCSP FSOM
Private practitioner, London
Director of Courses in Orthopaedic Medicine and Injection Therapy,
Orthopaedic Medicine Seminars and the Association of Chartered Physiotherapists in
Orthopaedic Medicine;
Fellow of Chartered Society of Physiotherapists, London, UK

With a contribution by
Steve Longworth

MB ChB MSc(Sports Medicine) MRCGP DM-SMED DPCR
Principal in General Practice, East Leicester Medical Practice,
Uppingham Road Health Centre, Leicester, UK

Foreword by
Gordon Cameron

MB ChB MRCGP DMsMED DCH FSOM
Principal in General Practice, Milton Surgery, Edinburgh, UK

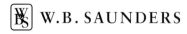 **W.B. SAUNDERS**

EDINBURGH   LONDON   NEW YORK   PHILADELPHIA   ST LOUIS   SYDNEY   TORONTO 2002

SAUNDERS
An imprint of Elsevier Science Limited

© Stephanie Saunders 1997, 2002
Illustrations © W. B. Saunders Company Limited 1997
Illustrations © Harcourt Publishers Limited 1999, 2002
Illustrations © Elsevier Science Limited 2002. All rights reserved.

The illustrations have been adapted from Ombregt, Bisschop, ter Veer,
and Van de Velde 1995 A system of orthopaedic medicine.
W. B. Saunders, London

First published 1997
Second edition 2002
Reprinted 2002

ISBN 0 7020 2632 8

British Library Cataloguing in Publication Data
A catalogue record for this book is available from the British Library

Library of Congress Cataloging in Publication Data
A catalog record for this book is available from the Library of Congress

Note
Medical knowledge is constantly changing. As new information
becomes available, changes in treatment, procedures, equipment and
the use of drugs become necessary. The authors and the publishers
have taken care to ensure that the information given in this text is
accurate and up to date. However, readers are strongly advised to
confirm that the information, especially with regard to drug usage,
complies with the latest legislation and standards of practice.

ELSEVIER SCIENCE
your source for books,
journals and multimedia
in the health sciences
www.elsevierhealth.com

The
publisher's
policy is to use
**paper manufactured
from sustainable forests**

Printed in China

Contents

Foreword

This is a book about the skill of using injections to treat patients with musculoskeletal pain. It will appeal to all of those who encounter such patients, but especially to general practitioners and physiotherapists.

I was involved as a contributor to the first edition of this book and at the time of publication there was a real sense of breaking new ground. Very few physiotherapists were skilled in injection therapy and those who were had learned in an ad hoc manner. How things have changed!

The authors of this new edition, Stephanie Saunders and Steve Longworth, have coordinated a very effective series of courses designed to teach injection techniques to experienced physiotherapists. Several hundred students have now graduated through the rigorous programme and passed the diploma exam that follows it. Far from being unusual, the ability to perform musculoskeletal injection is moving towards becoming a core part of physiotherapy practice. Credit for this lies with the authors and with those who have worked alongside them — notably ACPOM, the Association of Chartered Physiotherapists in Orthopaedic Medicine.

In the first edition of the book we tried to apply the 'keep it simple' principle. This edition picks up where its predecessor left off. The layout is logical, easy to follow and designed to be accessible at a glance. Readers who used and enjoyed the previous edition will find much that is familiar, but many improvements have been made. The opening chapters have been substantially expanded both in scope and content and are now lavishly referenced to reflect current research. The section on evidence-based practice is particularly welcome. New chapters covering injection techniques for spinal pain have been included, and the book is now truly a textbook rather than simply an instruction manual. All of this has been achieved without compromising the clarity of thought and illustration.

Both Stephanie Saunders and Steve Longworth are skilled practitioners but, more than that, they are excellent teachers and communicators. Their hard work and attention to detail in creating this book is clearly visible and without doubt this new edition is a worthy successor to the first. I recommend it wholeheartedly.

Edinburgh 2001   Gordon Cameron

Acknowledgements

An immense amount of time, effort and energy goes into the production of even a small textbook such as this, and I have been helped in making this second edition by an excellent team of people. No book is perfect, however.

My thanks go first to my colleague Dr Steve Longworth for his enormous enthusiasm in ensuring that his contribution was as up to date and evidence based as possible. Dr Gordon Cameron, who co-produced the first edition has always been most supportive and has kindly written a foreword to this edition.

Lynne Gardner, my secretary, has cheerfully coped with computer disasters and constant rewriting, and the Scottish team at Harcourt have been unfailingly helpful – through firm on deadlines!

Nick, my son, bravely exposed his body to many needles for the photographs, and the rest of the family have put up with laptops on holidays and instant meals at home.

I thank all my colleagues for encouraging me to write this book, my patients for allowing me to try different approaches, my students for constantly questioning my beliefs, and Dr James Cyriax, who taught me generously in his time.

Twickenham 2001   Stephanie Saunders

Preface

Steroid drugs have had a bad press in recent years. Many members of the public are worried about them and this fear is sometimes shared by those in the medical and paramedical professions. If injection therapy is used properly, however, the potential benefits vastly outweigh the possible side-effects.

The art of good injection therapy is to place the appropriate amount of the appropriate drug at the appropriate time into the exact site of the affected tissue. This means that the clinician practising injection therapy must possess a high level of diagnostic and technical skill.

PROBLEMS WITH INJECTION THERAPY ARISE WHEN:

- an *inappropriate drug* is chosen

- *too large a dose* is used

- injections are given *too frequently*

- the drug is put into the *wrong tissue*

- *poor injection technique* allows the spread of drugs to adjacent tissues

- insufficient attention is directed to the *cause of the lesion*

- no regard is given to *aftercare and rehabilitation.*

THE EVIDENCE BASE FOR INJECTION THERAPY

Despite the fact that injectable steroids have been around for more than 50 years, with a wealth of anecdotal evidence of their efficacy, there are few definitive studies of their application in joint and soft-tissue lesions[1-3], and few studies comparing injection therapy with other treatments[4-8]. This is even more astonishing given that steroid injection is the single commonest therapeutic intervention in rheumatological practice[9]. Consequently there are few facts and lots of opinions (most of them dogmatic and contradictory) about diagnosis, which lesions to treat, optimal steroid choice, steroid dosages, injection techniques, injection intervals and frequency, etc[9, 10-20].

Guidelines for physiotherapists are available[21] and, indeed, injection therapy administered by a physiotherapist has been shown to be part of a very effective way of managing orthopaedic[22] and rheumatology[23] outpatients and patients in the community with musculoskeletal lesions[24]. Extended Scope Practitioners (orthopaedic physiotherapy specialists) have been shown to be as effective as orthopaedic surgeons and to generate lower initial direct hospital costs[25].

The challenge for all clinicians delivering injection therapy is to seek and apply the best possible evidence-based treatments and hopefully, where evidence is lacking, to become involved in research that will provide that evidence.

See Appendix 2 for website addresses

Section 1

Guidelines and procedures

THE DRUGS

CORTICOSTEROIDS

The commonly used injectable steroids are synthetic analogues of the adrenal glucocorticocoid hormone cortisol (hydrocortisone), which is secreted by the innermost layer (zona reticularis) of the adrenal cortex. Cortisol has many important actions, including effects on protein and glucose metabolism, but it has also anti-inflammatory activity which is mediated by effects on polymorph and macrophage migration and suppression of the immunological response of lymphocytes[26,27].

When they were first administered systemically in the 1940s steroid drugs were hailed as the new 'universal panacea', but it soon became apparent that there were major side-effects that greatly limited their systemic use[28]. In 1951 Hollander in the USA reported the first use of local hydrocortisone injections for arthritic joints[29]. In 1967 triamcinolone hexacetonide (Lederspan) was introduced[30]. Virtually insoluble steroid suspensions are used because intra-articular soluble steroids will rapidly clear into the systemic circulation. The suspensions work by minute quantities of the active drug dissolving off the surface of the crystals while in contact with the inflamed tissue[28]. In joints, the steroid is taken up by the synovial cells, then gradually absorbed into the blood and cleared[1,31].

Corticosteroids exert their many effects on the cells involved in the immune and inflammatory responses primarily by modulating the transcription of a large number of genes. They act directly on nuclear steroid receptors to control the rate of synthesis of mRNA[32]. However, they also influence the mechanisms by which proteins are synthesized, and thereby affect the production of a wide range of pro-inflammatory mediators including cytokines[33] and other important enzymes.

RATIONALE FOR USING STEROID INJECTIONS

We know surprisingly little about the precise pharmacological effects of corticosteroids when they are injected directly into joints and soft tissues[34]. Local steroid injections are thought to work by:

- *Suppressing inflammation* in inflammatory systemic diseases such as rheumatoid or psoriatic arthritis, gout, etc[28,31,34–36].

- *Suppressing inflammatory flares* in degenerative joint disease[31,32,37–40]. The classic distinction between osteoarthrosis and osteoarthritis is not helpful, and there are no reliable clinical features which can tell us how much 'osis' (wear and tear) and how much 'itis' (inflammation) is contributing to a particular symptomatic joint[40]. Often, the only way to find out is to treat it.

- *Breaking up* the inflammatory *damage – repair – damage* vicious cycle which is postulated to set up a continuous low-grade inflammatory response, inhibiting tissue repair and sound scar formation, while forming adverse adhesions[41,42]. There is little direct evidence to support this, however.

- Possibly a direct *chondroprotective effect* on cartilage metabolism or other effects not related to anti-inflammatory activity of the steroids[32,43,44]

The precise role of inflammation in 'tendinitis' is the subject of considerable debate, and many authors prefer the terms 'tendinosis' or 'tendinopathy' to describe the pathological changes[45–48]. The pain may not be due to inflammation (tendinitis) or structural disruption of the tendon fibres (tendinosis), but the stimulation of nociceptors by chemicals released from the damaged tendon[49]. Corticosteroids (and possibly local anaesthetics) may affect the release of noxious chemicals and/or the long-term behaviour of local nociceptors.

CORTICOSTEROIDS USED FOR JOINT AND SOFT-TISSUE INJECTION

• Triamcinolone acetonide
'*Adcortyl*' (10 mg/ml – dilute)
'*Kenalog*' (40 mg/ml – strong)

Throughout the book we recommend Kenalog for ease of administration. This drug can be used in very small quantities so is ideal for small areas. Adcortyl may be used for larger joints and bursae. The duration of action is approximately 3 weeks.

• Methylprednisolone acetate
'*Depo-Medrone*' (40 mg/ml – strong)

May give more post-injection pain than other steroids[51]. Also comes in a fixed-dose combination with a local anaesthetic, Depo-Medrone (40 mg) with Lidocaine (10 mg/ml) in 1 ml and 2 ml vials, which we do not recommend.

• Hydrocortisone
'*Hydrocortistab*' (25 mg/ml – very weak)

Very soluble – the shortest duration of action of the steroids mentioned here[52]. We recommend its use particularly for superficial injections in thin, dark-skinned females, where there may be risk of depigmentation or local fat atrophy[53].

EQUIVALENT ANTI-INFLAMMATORY DOSES

4 mg of Triamcinolone or Methylprednisolone is equal to 20 mg of hydrocortisone.

SIDE-EFFECTS OF STEROID INJECTION

Systemic side-effects
- *Facial flushing*[36] is probably the commonest side-effect, occurring in from 5% of patients[1] to less than 1%[31]. It comes on within 24–48 hours after the injection and lasts 1–2 days.

Table 1 Common steroid preparations

Drug	Dose	Potency	Manufacturer
Short-acting	25 mg/ml	+	
Hydrocortisone acetate	1 ml		Knoll Pharma
(Hydrocortistab)	AMPOULES		
Intermediate-acting	40 mg/ml	+ + + +	
Methylprednisolone	1 ml, 2 ml, 3 ml		Upjohn
(Depo-Medrone)	VIALS		
Triamcinolone acetonide	10 mg/ml		Squibb
(Adcortyl)	1 ml AMPOULES		
	5 ml VIALS		
(Kenalog)	40 mg/ml		Squibb
	1 ml VIALS		
Long-acting		+ + + + + + +	
Dexamethasone	4 mg/ml	+ + + + + + +	MSD
(Decadron)	2 ml VIALS		

- *Uterine bleeding* (pre- and post-menopausal) may occur[4,54]. The mechanism is unknown (ovulation may be inhibited)[34]. In post-menopausal women this then creates a difficult dilemma – do you assume the bleeding is related to the injection, or should you investigate to exclude other, potentially serious, causes of post-menopausal bleeding? If this complication occurs it must always be taken seriously.

- *Deterioration of diabetic glycaemic control.* Diabetic patients must be warned about this possible temporary side-effect. There is also suppression of the hypothalamic – pituitary axis[55] following the intra-articular and intramuscular injection of corticosteroids[31,56], but at the doses and frequencies used in our approach to injection therapy this appears to be of no significant clinical consequence[57], therefore we do not issue patients with a steroid card after injection. Greater systemic absorption occurs if a given steroid dose is injected into several joints, presumably due to the greater synovial surface area available for drug transfer[31].

- *Significant falls in the ESR and CRP levels* (mean fall of about 50%). Intra-articular corticosteroid injections can cause this in patients with inflammatory arthritis and this effect can last for up to 6 months. This needs to be taken into account when using these blood tests to assess the response of patients to disease-modifying drugs like salazopyrin and methotrexate[58].

- *Other rare side-effects* from local steroid injection treatment include *pancreatitis* (patient presents with abdominal pain and the serum amylase is raised), *nausea, nerve damage, injection of the wrong drug, dysphoria* (emotional upset) or *posterior subcapsular cataracts*[5,31,34,67].

- *Anaphylaxis.* Severe anaphylactic reactions to local anaesthetic injections are rare, but can be fatal[59–61]. Anaphylactic reactions to locally injected corticosteroids are very rare but can occur[1]. They may be a reaction to the stabilizers the drug is mixed with rather than the steroid drug itself[57].

Table 2 Side-effects of steroid injection therapy

Systemic side-effects	Local side-effects
Facial flushing	Post-injection flare of pain
Menstrual irregularity	Skin depigmentation
Impaired diabetic control	Subcutaneous atrophy
Emotional upset	Bleeding/bruising
Hypothalamic–pituitary axis suppression	Steroid 'chalk'
Fall in ESR/CRP	Soft-tissue calcification
Anaphylaxis (very rare)	Steroid arthropathy
	Tendon rupture/atrophy
	Joint/soft-tissue infection

Consider carefully before giving corticosteroid injections to pregnant or breastfeeding women, even though some authorities recommend them for carpal tunnel syndrome during pregnancy[62]. There is no evidence that you will harm a woman or her baby, but pregnancy and childbirth are highly emotive, and if the mother has a difficult delivery or a baby with an abnormality she may try to blame your injection.

Local side-effects

Most local side-effects occur when too large a dose, in too large a volume, is injected too often. Subcutaneous placing of the steroid and using a bolus technique in tendons must be avoided.

- *Post-injection flare of pain.* The quoted figures are from about 2% to 10%[63,64], but this is well in excess of our own experience. When it does happen it is usually after a soft-tissue injection, and rarely follows joint injection[64]. It may be a reaction to the steroid's microcrystalline suspension and must always be distinguished from sepsis[28,31,36]. There may be more frequent post-injection flare with methylprednisolone, and this may have more to do with the vehicle or preservative in the drug than with the steroid itself[57].

  Multidose vials of Xylocaine contain *parabens* as a preservative. Many steroids will precipitate when added to it and this precipitate may be responsible for post-injection flare of pain or 'steroid chalk' (see below). Parabens may also be responsible for some allergic reactions to local injections. Single-dose vials of lignocaine do not contain parabens.

- *Subcutaneous atrophy* and/or *skin depigmentation*[31,65]. This is more likely to occur when superficial lesions are injected, especially in dark-skinned patients[53,66]. Take care not to allow injected drugs to reflux back through the needle tract–pressure around the needle with cotton wool when withdrawing may help. In thin dark-skinned women especially, it may be preferable to use hydrocortisone for superficial lesions. They must always be advised of the possibility of this side-effect, and the fact recorded in the notes.

- *Bleeding* or *bruising* may occur at the injection site.

- *Rare side-effects* include *nerve damage* (severe pain and 'electric shocks' if you needle a nerve), *transient paresis* of an extremity (from an inadvertent motor nerve block) and *needle fracture*[5,31,34,67].

- *Steroid 'chalk'* or *'paste'* may be found on the surface of previously injected tendons and joints during surgery. Suspension flocculation, resulting from the mixture of steroid with a local anaesthetic containing preservative, may be responsible. The clinical significance of these deposits is uncertain[31].

- *Soft-tissue calcification.* Corticosteroid injections into osteoarthritic interphalangeal joints of the hand may result in calcification or joint fusion, possibly because of pericapsular leakage of steroids due to raised intra-articular pressure[68]. No deleterious effects have been ascribed to this calcification.

- *Steroid arthropathy* is a well known and much feared complication of local injection treatment – it is also largely a myth[69]. Evidence exists that in many instances injected steroid can be chondro-protective rather than destructive[31,43], but the information from animal models about whether steroids damage or protect joints is contradictory[70]. There is good evidence linking prolonged high-dose *oral* steroid usage with osteonecrosis, but almost all the reports linking injected steroids with accelerated non-septic joint destruction are anecdotal, and mainly relate to joints receiving huge numbers of injections[69]. A reasonable guide[71] is to give injections into the major joints in the lower limbs at no less than 3–4 month intervals, although this advice is based on consensus rather than evidence[72]. Reports of Charcot-like accelerated joint destruction after corticosteroid injection in human hip osteoarthritis may reflect the disease itself rather than the treatment[31,73].

- *Tendon rupture*[74–77] or *atrophy*[78] is probably minimized by careful attention to technique, i.e. withdraw the needle a little if an unusual amount of resistance is encountered[74], and use a peppering technique at the enthesis with the smallest dose and volume of steroid that is effective[79]. The whole issue of steroid-associated tendon rupture is controversial[75–77], disputed[80], anecdotal[74], and not well supported in the literature[2,76], although it is widely accepted that the repeated injection of steroids into load-bearing tendons carries the risk of tendon rupture[81]. The current climate of opinion among consultants in rheumatology and sports medicine is against steroid injection into and around the Achilles tendon. It is advisable to image first (MRI or ultrasound) to confirm that it is a peritendinitis with no tendinopathy (degenerative change with or without tears in the body of the tendon). The patient should rest from provocative activity for 6–8 weeks[75] (consider putting the keen athlete into a walking cast), and return to it gradually after a graduated programme of stretching and strengthening.

- *Joint sepsis*[82] is the most feared complication of steroid injection treatment, but it is a rarity occurring in only one in 17 000–77 000 patients when performed as an 'office' procedure[31,68,83,84]. Prompt recognition is essential to prevent joint destruction, although diagnosis may be delayed by being mistaken for post-injection flare or exacerbation of the underlying arthropathy[85]. A case report by the Medical Defence Union highlighted a patient who developed septic arthritis following a steroid injection into the shoulder joint by her GP. The opinion of two experts was that infection is a rare hazard of the procedure, for which the GP should not be blamed[86].

- *Soft-tissue infections* can also occur after local injection treatment.

Most joint infections probably occur by haematogenous spread, rather than by direct inoculation of organisms into the joint. Steroid injection may create a local focus of reduced immunity in a joint, thus rendering it more vulnerable to blood-borne spread, rather than by introduction of organisms on the needle. Rarely, injection of contaminated drugs or hormonal activation of a quiescent infection may be to blame[82,85].

All cases of suspected infection following injection must be promptly admitted to hospital for diagnosis and treatment[82]. To avoid injecting an already infected joint have a high index of suspicion in patients with RA[87], elderly OA patients with an acute monarthritic flare (especially hip) and patients with coexistent infection elsewhere, e.g. chest, urinary tract and skin, especially the legs. Visualize and dip-stick the urine and check the ESR[88].

In the largest series of bacterial isolates reported from UK patients with septic arthritis, the commonest organisms were *Staphylococcus aureus* and *Streptococci* species. Others were *E. coli, Haemophilus influenzae, Salmonella* species, *Pseudomonas* species and *Mycobacterium tuberculosis*[89]. *M. tuberculosis* may be particularly difficult to diagnose, and may require the study of synovial biopsy samples[85].

Infection was most common in children and the elderly. Underlying risk-factors were reported in one fifth of cases, the most frequent being a prosthetic joint (11%). Others included haematological malignancy, joint disease or connective-tissue disorder, diabetes, oral steroid therapy, chemotherapy, presence of an intravenous line, intravenous drug abuse and post-arthroscopy[89]. Some surgeons deprecate the routine use of intra-articular steroids following arthroscopy for OA knee because of a perceived increased risk of infection following this procedure[70]. Steroid injection may also delay the presentation of sepsis by 6–12 days[70].

In a large prospective study carried out in an orthopaedic outpatient department complications of injection therapy were recorded in 672 patients receiving 1147 injections[64]. Just under 12% of patients (7% of injections) had any side-effect, but almost all of these were transient. Only four patients had subcutaneous atrophy at the injection site and these were all tennis elbow injections in females; the steroid dose was 4 times the dose we recommended. The commonest side-effect was post-injection pain but methylprednisolone was used which we believe causes more pain when injected into soft tissues than triamcinolone. When the data is reanalysed, 12% of the patients receiving periarticular injections had post-injection pain, but only 2% of those with intra-articular injections. Other side-effects were bleeding and fainting or dizziness.

Altogether, corticosteroids are remarkably safe. If one compares them to oral non-steroidal anti-inflammatory drugs, the justification for using the minimum effective dose of injectable steroid in the correct place with appropriate aftercare becomes obvious.

Table 3 Numbers needed to harm for patients prescribed an oral NSAID > 2 months	
Number	Harm caused
1 in 5	Endoscopic ulcer
1 in 70	Symptomatic ulcer
1 in 150	Bleeding ulcer
1 in 1200	Die from bleeding ulcer

Figures taken from Tramer et al[90]

LOCAL ANAESTHETICS

These membrane-stabilizing drugs act by causing a reversible block to conduction along nerve fibres. The smaller nerve fibres are more sensitive, so that a differential block may occur where the small fibres carrying pain and autonomic impulses are blocked, sparing coarse touch and movement[91].

Following most regional anaesthetic procedures, maximum arterial plasma concentrations of local anaesthetic (LA) develop within about 10–25 minutes[91]. This has implications for outpatient practice when significant volumes of LA are injected.

RATIONALE FOR USING LA

- *Diagnostic:* confirms diagnosis and correct placement of solution[92]. Sometimes even the most experienced practitioner will be unsure exactly which tissue is at fault. In this situation, inject a small amount of LA into the most likely tissue, wait a few minutes, and re-examine. If the pain is relieved then the source of the problem has been identified, and further treatment can be accurately directed.

- *Analgesic:* although the effect is temporary, it can make the overall procedure less unpleasant for the patient, break the pain cycle (by reducing nociceptive input to the 'gate' in the dorsal horn), and increase the confidence of the patient in the clinician, the diagnosis and the treatment. In one study, pain inhibition was better with bupivacaine than lidocaine during the first 6 hours, obviously because of its longer half-life; in later evaluations no differences in outcomes were observed[93]. In another study, bupivacaine was superior to lidocaine at 2 weeks, but not at 3 and 12 months[94]. Some practitioners inject a mixture of short- and long-acting LA in order to obtain the immediate diagnostic effect and more prolonged pain relief.

- *Dilution:* the internal surface area of joints and bursae is surprisingly large, due to the highly convoluted synovial lining with its many villae, so increased volume of the injected solution helps to spread the steroid around these structures. Distension is not required at entheses, so use the smallest volume that is practicable (distension in tendons by bolus injection of a relatively large volume of solution may physically disrupt the tendon fibres and compress the relatively poor arterial supply).

- *Distension:* a beneficial volume effect in joints and bursae may be physical stretching of the capsule or bursa with physical disruption of adhesions[95,96].

COMMONLY USED LOCAL ANAESTHETICS

The drugs most commonly used for joint and soft-tissue injection are:

- **Lidocaine Hydrochloride** (also known as lignocaine, brand name 'Xylocaine'). The most widely used LA, it acts more rapidly and is more stable than others. The duration of block is about half an hour.

- **Bupivacaine** (brand name 'Marcain'). It has a slow onset of action (about 30 min for full effect) but the duration of block is up to 8 hours. It is the principal drug for spinal anaesthesia in the UK and is *not advised* for routine outpatient clinic use.

- **Prilocaine** has low toxicity similar to lignocaine but is not as commonly used. **Procaine** is now seldom used. It is as potent as lignocaine but with shorter duration of action.

N.B. Lidocaine and Marcain are also manufactured with added adrenaline (which causes *vasoconstriction* when these drugs are used for skin anaesthesia, and so prolongs the LA effect). *DO NOT* inject these drugs into joints or soft-tissue lesions (the Xylocaine is clearly marked in red that it has adrenaline added).

Recommended maximum doses are given in Table 4. In practice, however, we suggest that much lower maximum doses are used – see Safety precautions, p. 13.

Table 4 Commonly used local anaesthetic drugs and maximum doses		
Drug	**Strength**	**Maximum dose and volume**
Lidocaine/Lignocaine	0.5% 5 mg/ml	200 mg 40 ml
	1.0% 10 mg/ml	200 mg 20 ml
	2.0% 20 mg/ml	200 mg 10 ml
Bupivacaine	0.25% 2.5 mg/ml	150 mg 60 ml
(Marcain)	0.5% 5 mg/ml	150 mg 30 ml

ADRENALINE (EPINEPHRINE)

Adrenaline is a vasoconstrictor which acts on the noradrenaline receptors and immediately physiologically reverses the symptoms of bronchospasm, laryngeal oedema and hypotension occurring in anaphylaxis or angioedema[97].

Adrenaline should always be at hand when infiltrating in case of an anaphylactic reaction to the LA. This is most conveniently carried in the form of an '*EpiPen*', which is an auto-injector for intramuscular use, pre-loaded with 1 mg/ml of adrenaline in 2 ml delivering a single dose of 0.3 ml (adrenaline 1:1000)[59–61].

OTHER INJECTABLE SUBSTANCES

SCLEROSANTS

Sclerotherapy[41] aims to strengthen inadequate ligaments by injecting them with an irritant to induce fibroblast hyperplasia. This causes soft-tissue inflammation, the opposite of steroid therapy. It is mostly used around the back, but may occasionally be indicated for a peripheral instability. In the USA this treatment is known as prolotherapy because it involves injecting a proliferant – a substance that causes fibro-blast proliferation. Sclerosing therapy was used by Hippocrates in the form of cautery at the shoulder to prevent recurrent shoulder dislocation. Sclerosing agents are mainly used to treat varicose veins, oesophageal varices and piles; their use in locomotor disorders has not caught on, despite evidence of their efficacy.

There are a large number of sclerosants, a common one being P2G which contains phenol, glucose and glycerine. Some prefer to use dextrose, which is potentially less neurotoxic although part of the pain-relieving effect may be due to a toxic action on nociceptors. Sclerosants are usually diluted with LA.

LUBRICANTS

In osteoarthritic (OA) joints, the synovial fluid's capacity to lubricate and absorb shock are typically reduced. This is partly due to a reduction in the size and concentration of hyaluronic acid (hyaluronan) molecules naturally present in synovial fluid, which produce a highly viscoelastic solution that is a lubricant at low shear and a shock absorber at high shear. A new approach in the management of knee OA is to inject hyaluronan or derivatives (hylans) into the joint[100].

Their mode of action is not clear – they stay in the joint cavity for only a few days. Perhaps they stimulate endogenous hyaluronan synthesis and/or reduce inflammation. Two preparations are licensed in the UK, with no evidence that one is superior. They are injected after the effusion is drained.

Hyalgan has the lower molecular weight of the two and is licensed as a medicinal product. It is injected once weekly for 5 weeks and is repeatable no more than 6-monthly. Synvisc has a higher molecular weight and is licensed as a medical device. It is injected once weekly for 3 weeks, repeatable once within 6 months, with at least 4 weeks between courses. Compared to placebo, both products produce a small reduction in pain that may last several months. The limited data available suggest that the products are as effective as continuous treatment with oral NSAIDs or intra-articular corticosteroid injections.

Guanethidine[101], radioactive materials[34,102], and even air[95,96] have been injected into joints to investigate their therapeutic potential.

DRUG NAMES

Rather confusingly, the same drug may go under different names in different countries. In 1992 the European Community decreed that in all member countries the World Health Organization's recommended international non-proprietary name (RINN) should be used exclusively. In the UK lignocaine has changed its name to lidocaine and adrenaline will become epinephrine. These names will change over at least 5 years, and there will be dual labelling during that time[103].

COSTS

All of the injectable drugs are remarkably inexpensive (UK prices 2000). One 1-ml ampoule of Adcortyl (10 mg of triamcinolone acetonide) costs £1.02, one bottle of Kenalog (40 mg) costs £1.70, while 10 ml of 1% lidocaine costs 42p. Compare this with the cost of a weak oral NSAID: a 1-month course of generic ibuprofen 400 mg tds costs £1.44 and of generic naproxen 500 mg bd (a more potent NSAID) costs £8.55 (and the brand name version Naprosyn costs £10.23)[97].

Injection therapy is cost-effective when compared to conventional physiotherapy[105].

DRUGS AND SPORT

Under the International Olympic Committee Medical Commission list of doping classes and methods (1998) local anaesthetics and corticosteroids are Class III drugs (subject to certain restrictions). They are permitted under restricted conditions and only if medically justified.

If you are not the team doctor and wish to use injection therapy for an athlete, we recommend that you discuss this with the team doctor. The athlete should be provided with a letter describing the rationale for treatment and the names and doses of drugs prescribed. If selected for a drugs test, the athlete should declare the treatment on the doping control form. Virtually insoluble corticosteroids (e.g. Lederspan) may be detectable months after the injection, although just how many months is difficult to say.

Beware the athlete who is taking performance-enhancing drugs. They will probably not admit it, but if they develop complications from the use of anabolic steroids they might blame your injection. Look out for the very muscular athlete with bad skin. Reviews of the use of injection therapy[39] and drug abuse in sport[81] can be found elsewhere.

SAFETY PRECAUTIONS

ASEPTIC TECHNIQUE

The following simple precautions should be taken to prevent any sepsis occurring:

- Use only pre-packed sterile disposable needles and syringes
- Use single-dose ampoules where possible
- Change needles after drawing up solution into the syringe
- Use domestically clean, dry hands – wet hands carry a greater risk of infection[104,106–109]
- Gloves are not normally necessary but in some countries are mandatory[110–111]
- Scrubbing up or wearing of gowns is not required
- Do not touch the skin after marking and cleansing the site
- Do not guide the needle with your finger
- When injecting a joint, aspirate to check that the fluid does not look infected.

ADVERSE REACTIONS

Toxic effects from corticosteroids and LAs are usually a result of excessive plasma concentrations. The main effects are excitation of the central nervous system (CNS) followed by CNS depression. Hypersensitivity to LA occurs very rarely[91,112] but the clinician must be prepared for any adverse reaction by taking the following precautions:

- Ask patient about any allergies to drugs, especially LAs, e.g. an allergic reaction to a dental injection. If in doubt, give a 1 ml intramuscular test-dose of LA
- Control amount of local anaesthetic given (see guidelines)
- Always aspirate before injecting, to check needle is not in a blood vessel
- Ask patient to wait for 30 min after the injection. Anaphylactic reactions begin rapidly, usually within 5–10 min of exposure. The time taken for the full reaction to evolve varies, but is usually 10–30 min[113].

SYNCOPE

A few people may faint, not as a reaction to *what* was injected, but to *being* injected – the result of fear, pain or needle phobia. Patients who express apprehension before having an injection should lie down for the procedure. You can be so intent upon placing the needle correctly that you miss the warning features of:

- pallor, sweating
- slight swaying

- lightheadedness, dizziness

- nausea

- tell you they are going to faint

- ringing in the ears

- vision 'going grey'

- bradycardia

- hypotension.

Syncope must be distinguished from an adverse drug reaction, and is treated by:

- reassuring the patient that they will shortly recover

- lying them down in the recovery position

- if loss of consciousness occurs, protecting airway and giving 35% oxygen.

Syncope may be accompanied by brief jerking or stiffening of the extremities, and may be mistaken for a convulsion by the inexperienced. Distinguishing a simple faint from a fit is helped by the presence of precipitating factors (painful stimuli, fear), and the other features described above. Incontinence is rare with syncope, and recovery of consciousness usually occurs within a minute[114].

ANAPHYLAXIS

A patient may be allergic to local anaesthetic and be unaware of it. A previous uneventful injection is not a guarantee that they will not be allergic this time, although it does provide some reassurance. The features may be any of the following[113]:

- flushing, itchy skin, urticaria

- nervousness

- nausea and/or vomiting

- feeling 'drunk' or confused

- abdominal pain

- profound hypotension

- tachycardia

- convulsions

- angio-oedema

- respiratory depression, bronchospasm causing severe respiratory difficulty

- sometimes a feeling of impending catastrophe.

Circulatory collapse, cardiac arrest and death may follow.

TREATMENT OF SEVERE ALLERGIC REACTIONS

- Maintain airway
- Summon help
- Administer adrenaline 1:1000 1 ml intramuscularly or subcutaneously
- Give 35% oxygen by mask
- Give cardiopulmonary resuscitation
- Establish intravenous access if necessary

ADVERSE REACTION REPORTING

In the UK any severe adverse reaction to any drug treatment should be reported to the Committee on Safety of Medicines (CSM) using the Yellow Card system. Yellow Card report forms can be found in the back of the British National Formulary (BNF). The Association of Chartered Physiotherapists in Orthopaedic Medicine (ACPOM) also has a reporting system for physiotherapists.

EMERGENCY SUPPLIES FOR THE TREATMENT ROOM

Have a supply of emergency equipment and medication available.

ESSENTIAL EMERGENCY KIT

- Disposable plastic airways
- An ambubag and mask for assisted ventilation
- Adrenaline 1:1000 strength
- Piriton 20 mg for injection
- Hydrocortisone for injection

ADDITIONAL EMERGENCY KIT FOR MEDICAL PERSONNEL

- Oxygen with masks and tubing
- A selection of IV canulae and fluid-giving sets
- Normal saline for infusion
- Plasma substitute for infusion

All drugs and fluids should be checked regularly to ensure they are not out of date.

HEALTH AND SAFETY

You should be vaccinated against Hepatitis B and have had a blood test to confirm immunity[115]. You may need a booster vaccination every 5 years. If in doubt, consult your doctor or hospital occupational health department.

Be aware of local policies on needle-stick injuries and what to do if you get one. There are national guidelines on the occupational exposure to HIV[116,117]. The best way to avoid a needle-stick injury is to be well organized and never to rush an injection.

ASPIRATION

If a joint effusion is present then aspiration is useful both diagnostically and therapeutically[72]. An effusion in a joint is known to result in loss of muscle strength (arthrogenic muscle inhibition), so physiotherapy is unlikely to be successful unless any effusion is suppressed[118,119]. In rheumatoid arthritis of the knee, aspiration of synovial fluid prior to steroid injection significantly reduces the risk of relapse[120].

Joint fluid may be loculated, very viscous and contain debris, all of which may prevent complete aspiration. With a small-bore needle it may be impossible to aspirate anything, so use at least a 21G or even a 19G needle. Moving the tip of the needle a few millimetres, or rotating it through 90 degrees may improve the flow into the syringe.

We recommend that disposable gloves are worn (to protect the clinician)[116] and towels be used (to protect the consulting room).

A 3-way connector between needle and syringe is useful to prevent having to disconnect the syringe if it is full but there is still fluid to aspirate. If this happens, the joint fluid tends to drip out of the disconnected needle (hence the need for something to catch the drips), so have another syringe ready to connect immediately. If the needle is left in the joint and the syringe is disconnected, the pressure between the inside and outside of the joint will equalise, and this may be why it is more difficult to aspirate.

After aspiration, immediately examine the fluid for colour, clarity and viscosity.

The clinical context will usually accurately predict the nature of the aspirate, which should always be sent for M/C+S (Microscopy, Culture and Sensitivity) to exclude crystal arthritis[121] and infection. Specifically request Z-N stain and await prolonged – usually 6 weeks – culture to exclude TB (immunosuppressed, Asians and alcoholics). Ideally, the fluid should be examined in the lab within 4 hours of aspiration. If analysis is delayed there will be a decrease in cell count, crystal dissolution, and artefacts will start to appear. Storage at 4°C will delay but not prevent these changes.

Although many laboratory tests may be performed on synovial fluid, only the white blood cell count (and percentage of polymorphonuclear lymphocytes), presence or absence of crystals, Gram stain, and bacterial culture (special cultures are needed if TB or fungal infection are suspected) are helpful[122].

Inoculation of the aspirate from joints and bursae into liquid media bottles (blood culture bottles) increases the sensitivity in the detection of sepsis[123,124]. *Staph. aureus* is the commonest organism in cases of septic arthritis and monosodium urate monohydrate crystals are present in gout.

WHAT THE ASPIRATE MIGHT BE AND WHAT TO DO

- *Frank blood.* Usually there is a history of recent trauma with the joint swelling up within hours. Aspiration gives pain relief, allows joint movement, and removes an irritant that causes synovitis. Blood often means a significant traumatic lesion so X-ray is mandatory. Haemarthrosis of the knee is due to anterior cruciate ligament (ACL) rupture in 40% of cases.

If there is a lipid layer on top of the blood this suggests intra-articular fracture. We advise that you do not inject a joint from which blood has been aspirated as there is unlikely to be a lesion that will respond, and injection may encourage further bleeding. There may also be rapid intravascular absorption from a bleeding surface. This view, however, has been challenged[39], and it is suggested that steroid injection following aspiration of a haemarthrosis may prevent a subsequent chemical synovitis and accelerate recovery. Recommended practice may change if and when more evidence becomes available. Further management depends on the cause of the haemarthrosis.

Rarely, haemarthrosis may be due to a bleeding disorder, anticoagulant treatment or from a vascular lesion in the joint, e.g. haemangioma.

- *Serous fluid of variable viscosity.* Normal or non-inflammatory synovial fluid is colourless or pale yellow (straw-coloured fluid). It contains few cells (less than 50 μl, mainly mononuclear) and little debris and therefore appears clear. It does not clot and is very viscous due to its high hyaluronic acid content. The 'drip test' forms a string 2–5 cm long before separating.

Should you aspirate and inject at the same time, or await the result of joint fluid analysis? This depends on the clinical context, appearance of the fluid, and experience of the clinician. If in doubt, DO NOT inject.

- *Serous fluid streaked with fresh blood.* This is not uncommon and is usually related to the trauma of the aspiration. It may occur at the end of the procedure when the tap becomes dry, or during the procedure if the needle tip is moved.

- *Xanthochromic fluid.* This is old blood which has broken down and appears orange in colour. Its presence implies old trauma.

- *Turbid fluid.* Inflammatory fluid tends to be less viscous than normal joint fluid, so it forms drops in the 'drip test'. It also looks darker and more turbid due to the increase in debris, cells and fibrin, and clots may form. It is impossible to say from the gross appearance what the inflammatory process is, so DO NOT inject, but await results of direct microscopy and culture studies.

- *Frank pus.* Rare in practice – patient is likely to be very ill and needs urgent admission. The aspirate would have a foul smell.

- *Other.* Uniformly milky-white fluid may result from plentiful cholesterol or urate crystals. Rice bodies are small shiny white objects composed of sloughed microinfarcted synovial villi. Greatly increased viscosity may be due to a recent steroid injection into that joint (or hypothyroidism).

UNEXPECTED ASPIRATION

Sometimes you may aspirate unexpected fluid which then contaminates the injection solution. Using gloves and towels, carefully disconnect the loaded syringe from the needle, taking care not to displace the needle and desterilize the tip of the syringe. Attach a fresh empty 10–20 ml syringe, lock it tightly onto the needle without displacement, and aspirate.

If the aspirate is 'suspect' do not inject. If it remains appropriate to inject, you can use the original solution, providing it is not too heavily contaminated and that the end of the syringe is kept sterile by attaching it to a sterile needle. If in doubt, draw up a fresh solution and be sure to lock syringe tightly onto the needle

Very rarely, you may puncture a blood vessel, e.g. an artery at the wrist in a carpal tunnel injection. Fresh bright-red arterial blood will pump into syringe, which should be withdrawn and firm pressure applied over the puncture site for several minutes.

ASPIRATING GANGLIA

In a study comparing aspiration of wrist ganglia with aspiration plus steroid injection, both treatments had a 33% success rate. Almost all ganglia which recurred after one aspiration did not resolve with further aspirations. After aspiration and explanation of the benign nature of ganglia, only one quarter of patients requested surgery[125].

INJECTION TECHNIQUE GUIDELINE

The following guidelines should be studied carefully before using any of the injection techniques.

In order to make the book easy to use we have simplified each technique and present only the essential facts. *Giving* injections is easy; it is the *selection* of the appropriate patient and injection that is difficult. The main points in the history and examination are given to aid the reader in this selection. While we suggest the use of Kenalog 40 (triamcinolone acetonide) and lidocaine throughout the book, any appropriate corticosteroid and local anaesthetic may be used.

HEADINGS

Each page covers one anatomical structure with the most common lesion found there.

CAUSES AND FINDINGS

Great care must be taken in the history and assessment. To aid in selection of appropriate patients, the common causes of the lesion and the main findings of the assessment are listed. When the patient has been examined, the different treatment options should be discussed, and the patient's consent to an injection gained (see Contraindications, p. 24).

EQUIPMENT AND DRUGS

The tables show the recommended size of syringe and needle, dosage and volume of corticosteroid and local anaesthetic, and total volume. These doses and volumes are usual for the average adult, but may be adapted for smaller or larger frames.

First decide on the strength (how many milligrams?) and the volume (how large is the structure to be injected?) required. Then choose a needle of the correct length to reach the structure, and a syringe of a size appropriate for the volume to be injected. All needles and syringes must be of single-use disposable type.

Syringes

Have available 1 ml, 2 ml, 5 ml, 10 ml and 20 ml syringes. Rarely a 50 ml syringe may be necessary for aspiration.

Use a small-bore 1 ml tuberculin syringe for small tendons and ligaments as the resistance of the structure can require a certain amount of pressure. Considerable back pressure may cause a larger syringe to blow off the needle and the clinician to be sprayed with the solution – an embarrassing situation.

Needles

Select the finest needle of the appropriate length to reach the lesion. Even on a slim person, it is often necessary to use a 75 mm or longer needle to successfully infiltrate deep structures such as the hip joint or psoas bursa. It is better to use a longer needle

Table 5 Needle sizes and colours most commonly used and universally available in the UK. Other countries may use different hub colours

Colour	Gauge	Width	Length
Orange	25G	0.5 mm	0.5 to 5/8 inch (13–20 mm)
Blue	23G	0.6 mm	1 to 1.25 inch (25–30 mm)
Green	21G	0.8 mm	1.5 to 2 inch (39–50 mm)
White	19G	1.1 mm	1.5 inch (40 mm)
Black	Spinal 21 or 22G	0.7–0.8 mm	3 inch (75 mm)

than you think necessary, than one which is too short which necessitates starting again. When injecting with a long fine spinal needle, it may be useful to keep the trochar in place to help control the needle as it passes through tissue planes.

Corticosteroid

Kenalog 40 (Triamcinolone acetonide with 40 mg steroid per ml) is the steroid we usually inject. In our experience it gives less afterpain in soft-tissue injections than Depo-Medrone (Methylprednisolone) and is equally effective.

Another advantage is that Kenalog can be used in both small and large areas, although where the total volume to be injected is large, the weaker solution, Adcortyl (Triamcinolone acetonide with 10 mg steroid per ml), can be used.

Local anaesthetic

Any suitable anaesthetic can be used. We suggest Lidocaine Hydrochloride used as follows:

- 2% Lidocaine up to maximum volume of 2 ml

- 1% Lidocaine for 2–5 ml

- dilute 1% with normal saline (0.9%) for injecting volumes larger than 5 ml.

Our recommended maximum doses are about half those published in pharma-cological texts[91], so well within safety limits. Occasionally Marcain is used where a longer anaesthetic effect is needed, but because of its longer half life we do not recommend it for these injections. Some practitioners like to mix a short- and long-acting anaesthetic.

Where any doubt exists about the possibility of the patient being allergic to local anaesthetic, *do not use it*. Volume may be obtained with normal saline if necessary.

Dosage and volume

The doses and volumes given below and in Table 6 are intended as guidelines only. They are governed by the size and age of the patient, the number of injections to be given and by clinical judgment.

Tendons and ligaments should have the minimum possible amount of volume and steroid inserted. A small volume avoids painful distension of the structure and the small dose minimizes risk of rupture. An average 'recipe' for most tendon lesions is 10 mg of steroid in total of 1 ml of local anaesthetic. Larger structures may require up to 20 mg of steroid in 2 ml volume.

Joints and bursae appear to respond best when sufficient fluid to slightly inflate the capsule or bursa is introduced. Possibly the slight distension 'splints' the structure or breaks down or stretches out adhesions.

Recommended maximum dosages and volumes in joint injections for an average-sized person are shown in Table 6. In a small patient the amounts are decreased. These volumes are well within safety limits and will not cause the capsule to rupture; for instance it is not unusual to aspirate over 100 ml of blood from an injured knee joint. In any case, the back pressure created by too large a volume would blow the syringe off the fine needle recommended, long before the capsule was compromised.

Table 6 Recommended maximum dosages and volumes for joint injections

	Dosage	Volume		Dosage	Volume
Shoulder	30 mg	10 ml	Hip	40 mg	5 ml
Elbow	20 mg	5 ml	Knee	40 mg	10 ml
Wrist, thumb	10 mg	2 ml	Ankle, foot	20 mg	5 ml
Fingers	5 mg	1 ml	Toes	10 mg	1 ml

ANATOMY

As an aid to identifying the structures, we have given tips for ways to remember individual sizes and to localize them, based on functional and surface anatomy. Where finger sizes are given, they refer to the *patient's* fingers, not the examiner's.

TECHNIQUE

This section describes in a logical sequence the procedure for administration of the solution. The steps are presented as bullet points for ease of execution.

Injections should *not* be painful. Skin is very sensitive, especially on the flexor surfaces of the body, and bone is equally so. Muscles, tendons and ligaments are less sensitive and cartilage virtually insensitive. Pain caused at the time of the injection is invariably the result of poor technique – *hitting* bone with the needle instead of *caressing* it. Afterpain can be caused by a traumatic periostitis because of damaging bone with the needle, or possibly by 'flare' caused by the type of steroid used. Success does not depend on a painful flare after the infiltration, although some patients do experience this. It is good practice to warn patients of possible afterpain and to ensure that they have painkillers available should they need them.

The secret of giving a reasonably comfortable injection depends on using the needle as an extension of the finger. The needle should be inserted *rapidly, perpendicular* to the *strongly stretched* skin and then passed gently through the tissue planes, feeding back information about the structures from the consistency of those tissues. The usual 'feel' of different tissues is as follows:

● Muscle – spongy, soft

● Tendon or ligament – fibrous, tough

● Capsule – often slight resistance to needle, like pushing through a balloon skin

- Cartilage – sticky, toffee-like

- Bone – hard and extremely sensitive.

Bursae and joint capsules are hollow structures requiring the solution to be deposited in one go – a *bolus technique*. No resistance to the introduction of fluid indicates that the needle tip is within a space. Chronic bursitis, especially at the shoulder, may result in loculation of the bursa. This gives the sensation of pockets of free flow and resistance within the bursa, rather like injecting a sponge.

Tendons and ligaments require a *peppering technique*. This helps to disperse the solution throughout the structure and to eliminate the possibility of rupture. The needle is gently inserted to caress the bone at the enthesis and the solution is then introduced in little droplets, as if into all parts of a sugar cube (see Figure below). Knowing the three-dimensional size of the structure is essential as this indicates the volume of fluid required and how much the needle tip has to be moved around. There is only one skin puncture; this is not multiple acupuncture.

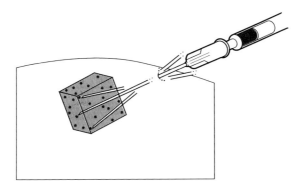

Tendons with sheaths. After inserting the needle perpendicular to the skin, lay the needle alongside the tendon within the sheath and introduce the fluid. Often a small bulge is observed contained within the sheath.

Blood vessels. Avoid puncturing a large blood vessel – if this occurs, apply firm pressure over site for 5 (vein) or 10 minutes (artery).

Aspiration. Check any aspirated fluid – if sepsis is suspected, aspirate with a fresh syringe and deposit in a sterile container for culture. Abandon the injection.

AFTERCARE

The ideal outcome is total relief of pain with normal power and range of motion. This does not always occur but when local anaesthetic is used there should be significant immediate improvement to encourage both patient and clinician that the correct diagnosis has been made and the injection accurately placed.

Explain the probable after effects of the injection to the patient. The relief of pain may be temporary, depending on the strength and type of anaesthetic used, and the pain may return when the effect of the anaesthetic wears off. Some patients describe this pain to be more than their original pain, but this is usually short-lived. This may be due to the flare effect which is thought to be caused by microcrystal deposition. It may also be that pain which comes back after a break may *appear* to be worse. Any after-pain can be eased by application of ice or taking simple analgesics.

The anti-inflammatory effect of the corticosteroid is not usually apparent until 24–48 hours after the infiltration and may continue for up to 3 months depending on the drug used.

Arrange to review the patient about a week or 10 days later, or sooner if the pain is severe or begins to return, as in acute capsulitis of the shoulder. Advise the patient on what to do and what to avoid. Usually joint conditions respond well to a programme of early gentle movement within the pain-free range.

If the symptoms were caused by overuse, the sporting or repetitive activity should not be engaged upon until the patient is symptom-free and a rehabilitation programme has corrected any defects.

Relative rest means that the normal activities of daily living can be followed – providing they are not painful. The patient should be encouraged to continue to do anything that is comfortable.

Once the symptoms have been relieved, the patient will usually need a few sessions of treatment for rehabilitation and prevention of recurrence. This may involve adaptation of movement patterns, correction of posture, stretching and/or strengthening regimes. The advice of a professional coach in their chosen sport or an expert in orthotics may also be required.

COMMENTS

In this section of each page we have listed the expected results of the treatment, complications that may occur and appropriate alternative approaches to treating the lesion described.

CONTRAINDICATIONS

ABSOLUTE CONTRAINDICATIONS TO INJECTION

- *local sepsis* over injection site
- suspicion of *infection* in the joint to be injected
- *sepsis elsewhere* (haematogenous spread; do not inject patients with a febrile illness
- *hypersensitivity to local anaesthetic* – steroid alone may be used

- *early trauma* – may induce further bleeding (unless aspirating blood)

- *haemarthrosis* – but this is disputed[39]; the pain relief obtained from aspiration can be dramatic; intra-articular fracture should be eliminated

- *prosthetic joint*

- *very unstable joint*

- *reluctant patient*

- *children* – injectable lesions are exceedingly rare under the age of 18 years and children spontaneously heal well; consider alternative diagnoses and diagnostic imaging

RELATIVE CONTRAINDICATIONS

- *diabetic* – greater risk of sepsis, blood sugar levels may rise for a few days or, rarely, longer

- *anticoagulated* – expect possible increased bleeding

- *bleeding disorder* – correct before injecting

- *immunosuppressed* – by disease (leukaemia, AIDS) or by drugs (systemic steroids)

- *psychogenic pain* – treatment may make the pain worse

- *severe anxiety* – signs of vagal overactivity leading to syncope

- *gut feeling* – when in doubt, do not inject

PREPARATION PROTOCOL

PREPARE PATIENT

- Discuss various treatment options, injection procedure and possible side-effects
- Obtain informed consent
- Place in comfortable sitting or lying position with injection site accessible

PREPARE EQUIPMENT

- Corticosteroid and local anaesthetic – check names, doses and expiry dates
- Syringe and needles for drawing up and infiltrating
- Spare syringe and sterile container for possible aspiration
- Alcohol swab, methylated spirit or iodine skin preparation
- Cotton wool and skin plaster

PREPARE SITE

- Identify structure and put skin under strong traction
- Mark site with clean finger nail, retracted end of ball-point pen, or needle guard
- Clean skin and allow to dry

ASSEMBLE EQUIPMENT

- Wash hands with suitable cleanser and dry well with disposable towel
- Clean rubber bungs of ampoules if not sterile and open vials
- Draw up steroid
- Draw up local anaesthetic from single-use vial
- Attach a fresh needle of correct size firmly to syringe

Use of gloves

Most clinicians in Britain do not use sterile gloves for injecting unless sepsis is suspected[9], but in some countries it is mandatory.

INJECTION TECHNIQUE FLOWCHART

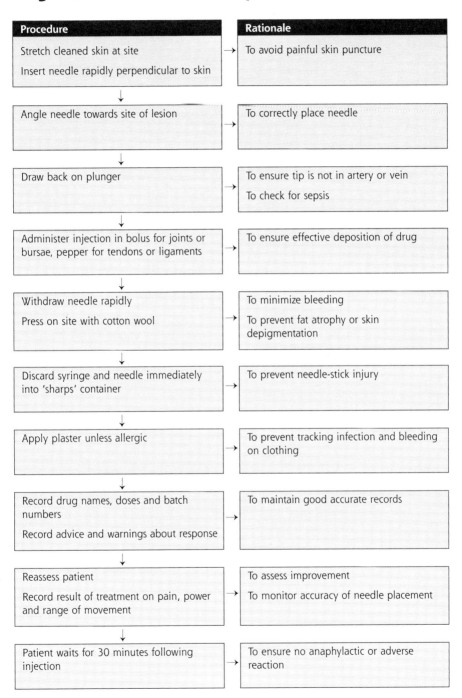

Procedure	Rationale
Stretch cleaned skin at site Insert needle rapidly perpendicular to skin	To avoid painful skin puncture
Angle needle towards site of lesion	To correctly place needle
Draw back on plunger	To ensure tip is not in artery or vein To check for sepsis
Administer injection in bolus for joints or bursae, pepper for tendons or ligaments	To ensure effective deposition of drug
Withdraw needle rapidly Press on site with cotton wool	To minimize bleeding To prevent fat atrophy or skin depigmentation
Discard syringe and needle immediately into 'sharps' container	To prevent needle-stick injury
Apply plaster unless allergic	To prevent tracking infection and bleeding on clothing
Record drug names, doses and batch numbers Record advice and warnings about response	To maintain good accurate records
Reassess patient Record result of treatment on pain, power and range of movement	To assess improvement To monitor accuracy of needle placement
Patient waits for 30 minutes following injection	To ensure no anaphylactic or adverse reaction

Section 2

Injection techniques: upper limb

SHOULDER JOINT

ACUTE OR CHRONIC CAPSULITIS – 'FROZEN SHOULDER'

Cause
Trauma
Osteoarthritis or rheumatoid arthritis
Idiopathic

Findings
Pain in deltoid area possibly radiating down to hand
Painful loss of: *most* passive lateral rotation with a hard end-feel
less passive abduction
least passive medial rotation

Equipment

Syringe	Needle	Kenalog 40	Lidocaine	Total volume
5 ml	21G 1.5–2" (0.8 × 40–50 mm)	30 mg	4.25 ml 1%	5 ml

Anatomy
The shoulder joint is surrounded by a large capsule and the easiest and least painful approach is posteriorly, where there are no major blood vessels or nerves. An imaginary oblique line running from the posterior angle of the acromion to the coracoid process anteriorly passes through the shoulder joint. The needle follows this line, passing through deltoid, infraspinatus and posterior capsule. Occasionally there is slight resistance when the needle passes through the capsule.

Technique
- Patient sits with arm held in medial rotation across waist
- Identify and mark posterior angle of acromion with thumb, and coracoid process with index finger
- Insert needle just below angle and push obliquely anterior towards coracoid process. End-point is when needle touches intra-articular cartilage
- Introduce fluid in a bolus

Aftercare
Maintenance of mobility with pendular and stretching exercises within the pain-free range, with stronger stretching when pain reduced.

Comments
The less the radiation of pain and the earlier the joint is treated, the more dramatic is the relief of symptoms. Usually one injection is successful in the early stages of the condition, but if necessary more can safely be given at increasing intervals of 1 week, 10 days, etc. Rarely the posterior approach is not effective, so then an anterior approach can be used. In this case, the arm is held in lateral rotation and the needle is inserted on the anterior surface between the coracoid process and the lesser tuberosity of the humerus and aimed posteriorly towards the spine of the scapular. The same dose and volume are used.

SHOULDER JOINT

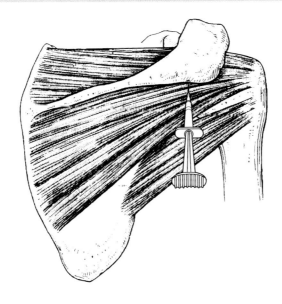

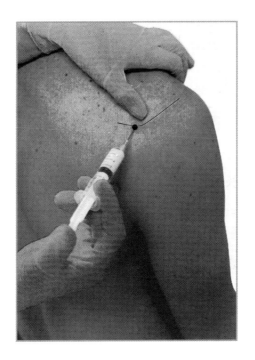

ACROMIO-CLAVICULAR JOINT

ACUTE OR CHRONIC CAPSULITIS

Cause
Trauma
Occasionally prolonged overuse

Findings
Pain at point of shoulder
Painful: end-range of all passive movements, especially full passive horizontal
        adduction
        occasional *arc* on active elevation

Equipment

Syringe	Needle	Kenalog 40	Lidocaine	Total volume
1 ml	25G 0.5″ (0.5 × 16 mm)	10 mg	0.75 ml 2%	1 ml

Anatomy
The acromio-clavicular joint line runs in the sagittal plane about a thumb's width medial to the lateral edge of the acromion. The joint plane runs obliquely medially and usually contains a small meniscus. Often a small step can be palpated where the acromion abuts against the clavicle, or a small V-shaped gap felt at the anterior joint margin.

Technique
- Patient sits supported with arm hanging by side to slightly separate the joint surfaces
- Identify lateral edge of acromion. Move medially about a thumb's width and mark joint line
- Insert needle angling medially about 30° and pass through capsule
- Deposit solution in a bolus

Aftercare
Relative rest for 1 week then gentle mobilizing exercises. Acutely inflamed joints are helped by the application of ice and taping to stabilize the joint.

Comments
Occasionally the joint is difficult to enter. Traction on the arm and peppering of the capsule with the solution while feeling for the joint space is recommended. The unstable joint may be helped by sclerosing injections or possibly surgery.

ACROMIO-CLAVICULAR JOINT

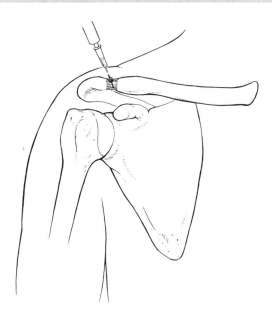

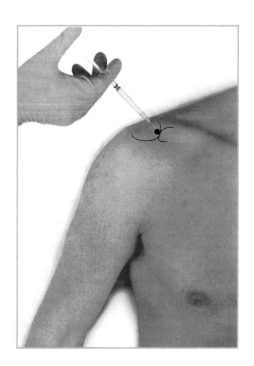

STERNO-CLAVICULAR JOINT

ACUTE OR CHRONIC CAPSULITIS

Cause
Trauma or overuse

Findings
Pain over sterno-clavicular joint
Painful: retraction and protraction of the shoulder
full elevation of the arm
clicking

Equipment

Syringe	Needle	Kenalog 40	Lidocaine	Total volume
1 ml	25G 0.5" (0.5 × 16 mm)	10 mg	0.75 ml 2%	1 ml

Anatomy
The sterno-clavicular joint contains a small meniscus which can sometimes give painful symptoms. The joint line runs obliquely laterally from superior to inferior and can be identified by palpating the joint medial to the end of the clavicle while the patient protracts and retracts the shoulder.

Technique
- Patient sits supported with arm in slight lateral rotation
- Identify and mark joint line
- Insert needle perpendicularly through joint capsule
- Deposit solution in bolus

Aftercare
Rest for a week followed by mobilization and a progressive postural and exercise regime.

Comments
Although not a common lesion, this usually responds well to one infiltration.

STERNO-CLAVICULAR JOINT

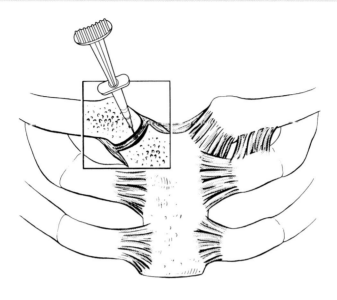

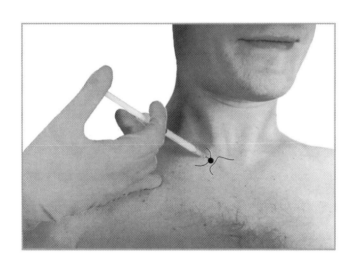

SUBACROMIAL BURSA

CHRONIC BURSITIS

Cause
Overuse

Findings
Pain in deltoid area
Painful: passive elevation and medial rotation
         resisted abduction and lateral rotation, often on release of resistance
         often, but not always, *arc* on active abduction

Equipment

Syringe	Needle	Kenalog 40	Lidocaine	Total volume
5 ml	23G 1.25″ (0.6 × 30 mm)	20 mg	4.5 ml 1%	5 ml

Anatomy
The bursa lies mainly under the acromion, but is variable in size and there may be more than one. Occasionally a tender area can be palpated around the edge of the acromion.

Technique
- Patient sits with arm hanging by side to distract humerus from acromion
- Identify and mark lateral edge of acromion
- Insert needle at mid-point of acromion and angle slightly upwards under acromion to full length
- Slowly withdraw needle while simultaneously injecting fluid in a bolus wherever there is no resistance. Sometimes the fluid causes visible swelling around the edge of the acromion

Aftercare
Relief of pain after one injection is usual but the patient must maintain retraction and depression of the shoulders and avoid elevation of the arm above shoulder level for 1 week. Taping the shoulder in retraction/depression is helpful. After this the patient commences resisted lateral rotation and retraction exercises and retraining of overarm activities in order to avoid recurrence.

Comments
This is the most common injectable lesion found in orthopaedic medicine – see Appendix 1. Results are usually excellent but the exercise programme must be maintained to prevent recurrence. In long-standing bursitis there is often loculation. In this case resistance is felt while injecting the solution, so the needle must be fanned around under the acromion in order to inject separate pockets of the bursa. The sensation is that of injecting a sponge. Occasionally calcification occurs within the bursa and hard resistance is felt. Infiltration with a large-bore needle and local anaesthetic may be helpful. Failing this, surgical clearance is recommended[123].

SUBACROMIAL BURSA

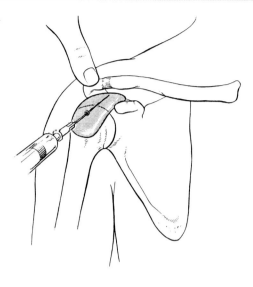

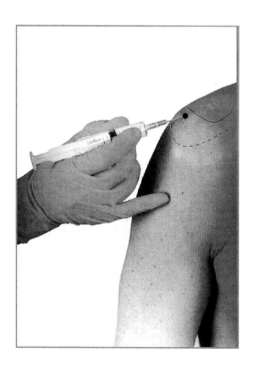

SUPRASPINATUS TENDON

CHRONIC TENDINITIS

Cause
Overuse

Findings
Pain in deltoid area
Painful: resisted abduction
          arc on active abduction

Equipment

Syringe	Needle	Kenalog 40	Lidocaine	Total volume
1 ml	25G 0.5" (0.5 × 16 mm)	10 mg	0.75 ml 2%	1 ml

Anatomy
The greater tuberosity of the humerus, into which the tendon inserts, lies in a direct line with the lateral epicondyle of the elbow. A line joining the two points passes through the tendon which is approximately the size of the middle finger at insertion into the superior facet.

Technique
- Patient sits supported with forearm medially rotated behind back, bringing the tendon forward, so it lies just anterior to the edge of the acromion
- Identify lateral epicondyle of the elbow, now facing anteriorly, and run finger up front of humerus to touch anterior edge of acromion. The greater tuberosity now lies immediately anterior with the tendon insertion in the hollow between the two bones. Mark this facet
- Insert needle perpendicularly through tendon to touch bone
- Pepper solution into tendon

Aftercare
Relative rest for 1 week then progressive exercise regime and postural control when symptom-free.

Comments
Supraspinatus tendinitis can occur on its own but is more commonly associated with subacromial bursitis. Always treat the bursa first and if some pain remains on resisted abduction, then the tendon can be infiltrated a week or so later.

Calcification can arise within the tendon and hard resistance can be felt with the needle. The symptoms often recur but it is worth attempting to break up the calcification with a large-bore needle and local anaesthetic. The results are variable. If symptoms persist a surgical opinion should be sought.

SUPRASPINATUS TENDON

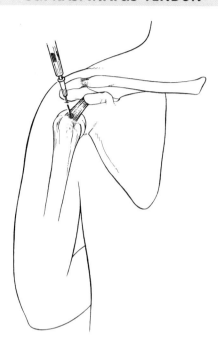

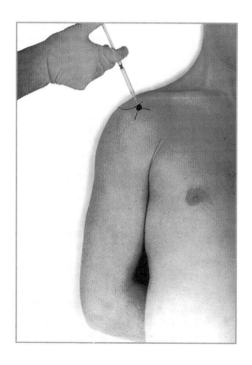

INFRASPINATUS TENDON

CHRONIC TENDINITIS

Cause
Overuse

Findings
Pain in deltoid area
Painful: resisted lateral rotation
         arc on active abduction

Equipment

Syringe	Needle	Kenalog 40	Lidocaine	Total volume
2 ml	23G 1.25″ (0.6 × 30 mm)	15–20 mg	1.25–1.5 ml 2%	1.5–2 ml

Anatomy
The infraspinatus and teres minor tendons insert together into the middle and lower facets on the posterior aspect of the greater tuberosity of the humerus. They are together approximately three fingers wide at the teno-osseous insertion.

Technique
- Patient sits with supported arm flexed to right angle and held in adduction and lateral rotation. This brings the posterior facets out from under the thickest portion of the deltoid and puts the tendon under tension running obliquely upwards and laterally
- Identify posterior angle of acromion. Tendon insertion now lies 45° inferior and lateral in direct line with lateral epicondyle of the elbow. Mark this spot on the two posterior facets
- Insert needle at mid-point of tendons at insertion. Pass through tendon and touch bone
- Pepper solution in two rows up and down into teno-osseous junction

Aftercare
Relative rest for 1 week then progressive exercise regime and postural correction when symptom-free.

Usually a painful arc is present which indicates that the lesion lies at the teno-osseous junction. Occasionally there is no arc when the lesion lies in the body of the tendon. In this case the needle is inserted more medially where there is often an area of tenderness, and the same technique applied.

Comments
The smaller patient is given the smaller amount of volume but for a large man, a greater volume and dose are required.

INFRASPINATUS TENDON

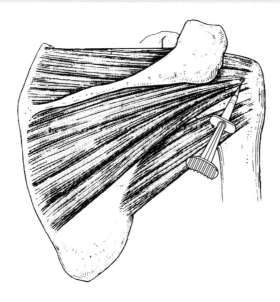

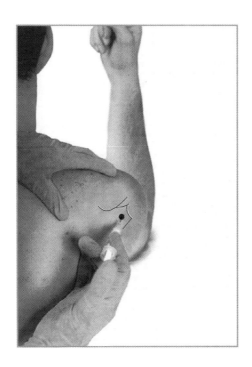

SUBSCAPULARIS TENDON AND BURSA

ACUTE OR CHRONIC TENDINITIS OR BURSITIS

Cause
Overuse or trauma

Findings
Pain in deltoid area or anterior to shoulder
Painful: resisted medial rotation
        arc on active abduction
        passive lateral rotation and full passive horizontal adduction (scarf test)

Equipment

Syringe	Needle	Kenalog 40	Lidocaine	Total volume
Tendon 1 ml Bursa 2 ml	23G 1–1.25″ (0.6 × 25–30 mm)	Tendon 10 mg Bursa 20 mg	Tendon 0.75 ml 2% Bursa 1.5 ml 2%	Tendon 1 ml Bursa 2 ml

Anatomy
The subscapularis tendon inserts into the medial edge of the lesser tuberosity of the humerus. It is approximately two fingers wide at its teno-osseous insertion and feels bony to palpation.

  The subscapularis bursa lies deep to the tendon in front of the neck of the scapula and usually communicates with the joint capsule of the shoulder. It is always extremely tender to palpation.

Technique
- Patient sits supported with arm by side and held in 45° lateral rotation
- Identify coracoid process. Move laterally to feel small protuberance of lesser tuberosity by passively rotating arm. Mark this spot on medial aspect of tuberosity
- Insert needle at mid-point of tuberosity angling slightly laterally. Touch bone at insertion
- Pepper solution into tendon insertion or deposit bolus deep to tendon into bursa

Aftercare
Relative rest for 1 week then progressive stretching and strengthening programme when pain-free.

Comments
Subscapularis bursitis and tendinitis are often difficult to differentiate. The bursa is implicated if there is more pain on the scarf test than on resisted medial rotation, and if there is even more than usual tenderness to palpation. They are often inflamed together and then both can be infiltrated at the same time by peppering the tendon first and then going through it to infiltrate the bursa.

SUBSCAPULARIS TENDON AND BURSA

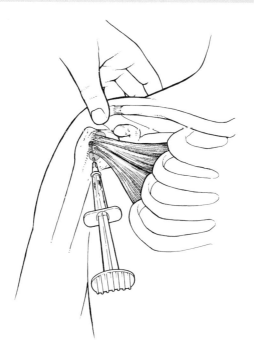

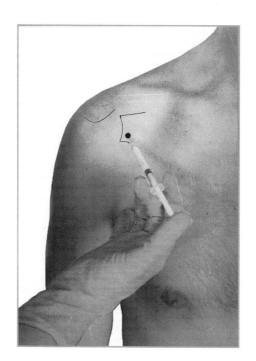

SUPRASCAPULAR NERVE

ACUTE OR CHRONIC CAPSULITIS – 'FROZEN SHOULDER'

Cause
Trauma
Osteoarthritis or rheumatoid arthritis
Idiopathic

Findings
Pain in deltoid area possibly radiating down to hand
Painful loss of: *most* passive lateral rotation with a hard end-feel
less passive abduction
least passive medial rotation

Equipment

Syringe	Needle	Kenalog 40	Lidocaine	Total volume
5 ml	21G 1.75″ (0.8 × 40 mm)	20 mg	4.5 ml 1%	5 ml

Anatomy
The suprascapular nerve passes through the suprascapular notch into the supraspinous fossa, passes laterally to curl around the neck of the spine of the scapula and ends in the infraspinous fossa. It supplies the supraspinatus and infraspinatus, and sends articular branches to the shoulder and acromio-clavicular joints. For this reason it is worth injecting here where intracapsular injection has not been successful.

Technique
- The patient sits supported with arm in neutral position
- Identify mid-point of spine of scapular and mark spot one finger cephalad and one finger lateral
- Insert needle perpendicular to suprascapular fossa and angle slightly laterally to touch bone
- Deposit solution as bolus

Aftercare
Mobility at the shoulder is maintained within pain-free range. Stretching and mobilization are started when pain permits.

Comments
A small randomized trial suggests that suprascapular nerve block is a safe and effective alternative treatment for frozen shoulder in primary care[126]. Some clinicians advise the use of a longer-lasting anaesthetic alone or with corticosteroid. This injection may also be useful in patients with rotator cuffs tears who are not fit for surgery.

SUPRASCAPULAR NERVE

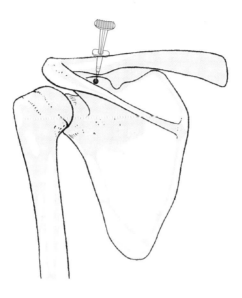

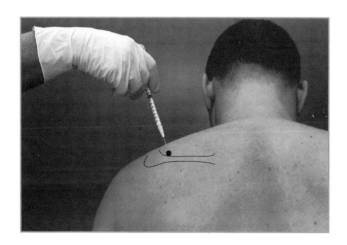

ELBOW JOINT

ACUTE OR CHRONIC CAPSULITIS

Cause
Trauma
Occasionally heavy overuse, e.g. fencing

Findings
Pain in and around elbow joint
Painful: passive limitation of *more* flexion
　　　　　less extension

Equipment

Syringe	Needle	Kenalog 40	Lidocaine	Total volume
2 ml	25G 0.5″ (0.5 × 16 mm)	20 mg	1.5 ml 2%	2 ml

Anatomy
The capsule of the elbow joint contains all three joints – the radio-humeral, radio-ulnar and humero-ulnar. The posterior approach above the top of the head of the radius is the safest and easiest.

Technique
- Patient sits with elbow supported at 45° of flexion
- Identify head of radius posteriorly and mark space between it and humerus
- Insert needle parallel to the top of the head of radius and penetrate capsule
- Deposit solution in a bolus

Aftercare
After a couple of days the patient should start increasing range of motion within the limits of pain using gentle stretching movements, and passive mobilization techniques are effective.

Comments
This is not a very common injection but may be useful after trauma.

If the cause of the symptoms is one or more loose bodies within the joint, the treatment is mobilization under strong traction. If the range is improved by this but the pain persists, an injection may be considered.

ELBOW JOINT

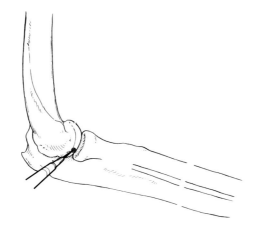

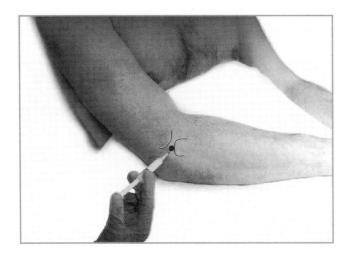

OLECRANON BURSA

ACUTE OR CHRONIC BURSITIS

Cause
Sustained compression or fall/direct blow onto elbow

Findings
Pain at posterior aspect of elbow joint
Painful: passive flexion and sometimes extension
              resisted extension
Tender area over bursa and occasionally obvious swelling

Equipment

Syringe	Needle	Kenalog 40	Lidocaine	Total volume
2 ml	23G 1″ (0.6 × 25 mm)	20 mg	1.5 ml 2%	2 ml

Anatomy
The bursa lies at the posterior aspect of the elbow and is approximately the size of a golf ball.

Technique
- Patient sits with supported elbow at right angle
- Identify and mark centre of tender area of bursa
- Insert needle into central area
- Deposit solution into bursa in a bolus

Aftercare
Relative rest for a week then resumption of normal activities avoiding leaning on elbow.

Comments
Occasionally a direct blow or fall may cause haemorrhagic bursitis, when the treatment should be immediate aspiration of all blood prior to the infiltration. Aspiration is always done first and if suspicious fluid is withdrawn, infiltration should not be given at the same time.

OLECRANON BURSA

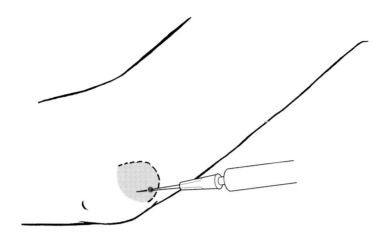

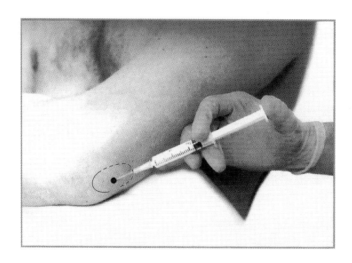

COMMON EXTENSOR TENDON

CHRONIC TENDINITIS – 'TENNIS ELBOW'

Cause
Overuse

Findings
Pain at lateral aspect of elbow
Painful: resisted extension of the wrist with elbow extended
        passive wrist flexion with ulnar deviation

Equipment

Syringe	Needle	Kenalog 40	Lidocaine	Total volume
1 ml	25G 0.5″ (0.5 × 16 mm)	10 mg	0.75 ml 2%	1 ml

Anatomy
Tennis elbow invariably occurs at the teno-osseous origin of the common extensor tendon at the elbow. The tendon arises from the anterior facet of the lateral epicondyle, which is approximately the size of the little finger nail.

Technique
- Patient sits with supported elbow bent at right angle and forearm supinated
- Identify and mark facet lying anteriorly on lateral epicondyle
- Insert needle in line with cubital crease perpendicular to the facet to touch bone
- Pepper solution into tendon

Aftercare
The patient rests the elbow for 10 days. Any lifting must be done only with the palm facing upward so that the flexors rather than the extensors are used, and the causal activity avoided. When resisted extension is pain-free, two or three sessions of deep friction with a strong extension manipulation are given to prevent recurrence. Stretching of the extensors and a strengthening programme is gradually started. If the cause was a racquet sport, the weight, handle-size and stringing of the racquet and the stroke should be checked.

Comments
Although the teno-osseous junction is the most common site, the lesion can occur in the body of the tendon, in the muscle belly and at the origin of the extensor carpi radialis longus. Ignore tender trigger points in the body of the tendon, present in everyone, and place the needle exactly at the very small site of the lesion.

   One injection usually suffices, but if symptoms recur, a second injection is given followed by the above routine a few days later. Alternatively, sclerosant injection can be used. Failing these, tenotomy may be performed. Depigmentation and/or subcutaneous atrophy may occur in thin females, especially those with dark skins, and they should be informed of this before giving consent.

COMMON EXTENSOR TENDON

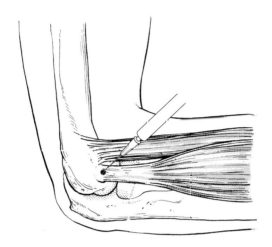

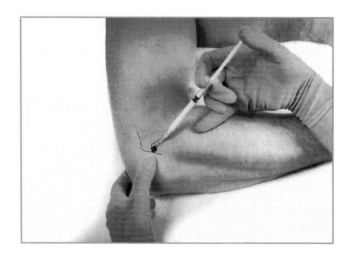

COMMON FLEXOR TENDON

CHRONIC TENDINITIS – 'GOLFER'S ELBOW'

Cause
Overuse

Findings
Pain at medial aspect of elbow
Painful: resisted flexion of wrist
           occasionally resisted pronation of elbow

Equipment

Syringe	Needle	Kenalog 40	Lidocaine	Total volume
1 ml	25G 0.5" (0.5 × 16 mm)	10 mg	0.75 ml 2%	1 ml

Anatomy
The common flexor tendon at the elbow arises from the anterior facet on the medial epicondyle. It is approximately the size of the little finger nail at its teno-osseous origin.

Technique
- Patient sits with supported arm extended
- Identify and mark anterior facet on medial epicondyle
- Insert needle perpendicular to facet and touch bone
- Pepper solution into tendon

Aftercare
Relative rest for 1 week then stretching and strengthening exercises.

Comments
Occasionally the lesion occurs at the musculo-tendinous junction. Infiltration at this point may not be as effective but deep friction can be successful.

COMMON FLEXOR TENDON

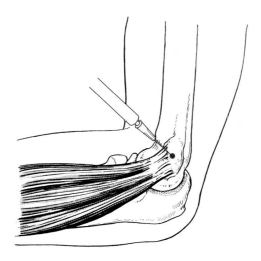

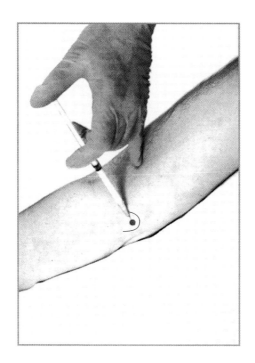

BICEPS TENDON INSERTION

CHRONIC TENDINITIS OR BURSITIS

Cause
Overuse

Findings
Pain at front of elbow
Painful: resisted flexion and supination of elbow
         plus passive extension and pronation of elbow if bursa affected

Equipment

Syringe	Needle	Kenalog 40	Lidocaine	Total volume
Tendon 1 ml Bursa 2 ml	23G 1.25" (0.6 × 30 mm)	Tendon 10 mg Bursa 20 mg	Tendon 0.75 ml 2% Bursa 1.5 ml 2%	Tendon 1 ml Bursa 2 ml

Anatomy
Although the biceps can be affected at any point along its length, the most usual site is its insertion into the radial tuberosity on the antero-medial aspect of the shaft of the radius. A small bursa lies at this point and can be inflamed together with the tendon or on its own.

    The insertion of the biceps is identified by following the path of the tendon distal to the cubital crease while the patient resists elbow flexion. The patient then relaxes the muscle and the tuberosity can be palpated on the ulnar side of the radius while passively pro- and supinating the forearm. The site is always very tender to palpation.

Technique
- Patient lies face down with arm extended and palm flat on table. Passively pronate forearm fully while keeping humerus still
- Identify and mark radial tuberosity two fingers distal to radial head
- Insert needle perpendicularly to touch bone
- Pepper solution into tendon or bolus into bursa, or both as necessary

Aftercare
Rest for 1 week before beginning graded strengthening and stretching routine.

Comments
Differentiation between bursitis and tendinitis is often difficult. If there is more pain on passive flexion and pronation of the elbow than on resisted flexion, together with extreme sensitivity to palpation, the bursa is more suspect. If in doubt, infiltrate the bursa first and assess a week later.

BICEPS TENDON INSERTION

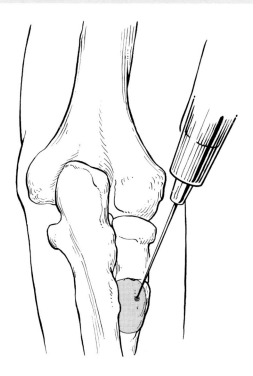

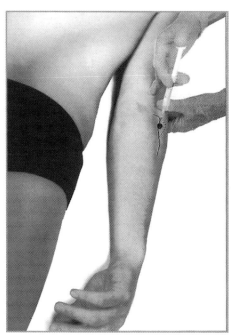

WRIST JOINT

ACUTE CAPSULITIS

Cause
Rheumatoid arthritis
Trauma

Findings
Pain in and around wrist joint
Painful: equal limitation of passive extension and flexion

Equipment

Syringe	Needle	Kenalog 40	Lidocaine	Total volume
2 ml	23G 1.25" (0.6 × 30 mm)	20 mg	1.5 ml 2%	2 ml

Anatomy
The wrist joint capsule is not continuous and has septa dividing it into separate compartments. For this reason it cannot be injected at one spot, but requires several points of infiltration.

Technique
- Patient places hand palm down
- Identify and mark mid-carpus proximal to hollow dip of capitate
- Insert needle at mid-point of carpus
- Deposit solution at different points across the dorsum of the wrist, both into the ligaments and also intracapsular where possible

Aftercare
The patient rests in a splint until the pain subsides and then begins gentle mobilizing exercises within the pain-free range.

Comments
This is not a common area for injection except in the patient with rheumatoid arthritis. Patients with other causes such as trauma, overuse or osteoarthritis usually respond well to a short period of pain-relieving modalities, medication and rest in a splint, followed by passive and active mobilization techniques.

WRIST JOINT

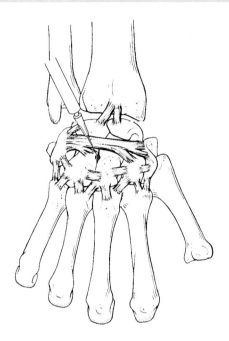

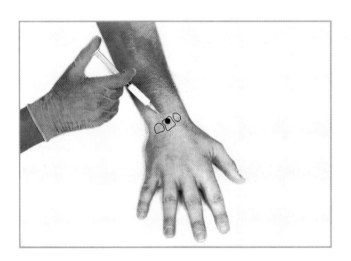

INFERIOR RADIO-ULNAR JOINT

CHRONIC CAPSULITIS OR ACUTE TEAR OF THE MENISCUS

Cause
Osteoarthritis or rheumatoid arthritis
Trauma

Findings
Pain at end of forearm on ulnar side
Painful: passive pronation and supination at end-range
          resisted flexion and ulnar deviation if meniscus torn

Equipment

Syringe	Needle	Kenalog 40	Lidocaine	Total volume
2 ml	25G 0.5″ (0.5 × 16 mm)	10 mg	1 ml 2%	1.25 ml

Anatomy
The inferior radio-ulnar joint is an L-shaped joint about a finger's width in length and includes the triangular cartilage which separates the ulnar from the carpus. With the palm facing downwards, the joint lies one third across the wrist just medial to the bump of the end of the ulnar. The joint line is identified by gliding the ends of the radius and ulnar against each other.

Technique
- Patient sits with hand palm down
- Identify and mark styloid process of ulnar
- Insert needle just distal to styloid aiming transversely towards radius and penetrate capsule
- Deposit solution in bolus

Aftercare
Rest for 1 week and avoidance of flexion/ulnar deviation activities. Mobilization with distraction can be effective in meniscal tears.

Comments
Tears of the cartilage are quite common, especially after trauma or fracture. In this case pain is found on full passive supination and flexion, and on resisted flexion in ulnar deviation. The most pain-provoking test is the scoop test – compressing the supinated wrist into ulnar deviation and scooping it in a semi-circular movement towards flexion. The patient often complains of painful clicking and occasionally the wrist locks. Mobilization helps relieve the pain but an injection can be given in the acute phase.

INFERIOR RADIO-ULNAR JOINT

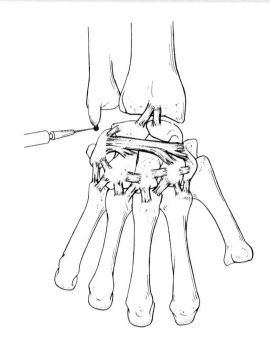

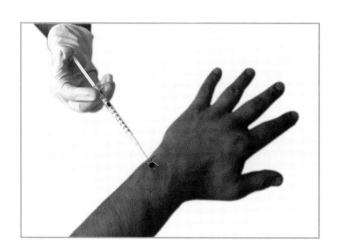

THUMB AND FINGER JOINTS

ACUTE OR CHRONIC CAPSULITIS

Cause

Overuse or trauma

Findings

Thumb: painful and limited passive adduction of thumb backwards behind hand
painful and limited passive extension

Fingers: painful and limited passive flexion at interphalangeal joints
painful and limited passive extension at distal phalangeal joints

Equipment

Syringe	Needle	Kenalog 40	Lidocaine	Total volume
1 ml	25G 0.5″ (0.5 × 16 mm)	Thumb 10 mg Fingers 5 mg	Thumb 0.75 ml 2% Fingers 0.5 ml 2%	Thumb 1 ml Fingers 0.75 ml

Anatomy

The first metacarpal articulates with the trapezium. The easiest entry-site is at the apex of the snuff-box on the dorsum of the wrist. The joint line is found by passively flexing and extending the thumb while palpating for the joint space between the two bones. The radial artery lies at the base of the snuff-box.

The distal thumb and finger joints can best be infiltrated from the medial or lateral aspect at the joint line.

Technique

- Patient rests hand in mid position with thumb up
- Identify and mark gap of joint space
- Insert needle perpendicularly into gap
- Deposit solution in a bolus

Aftercare

Patient begins gentle active and passive mobilizing exercise within pain-free range and is advised against overuse of the thumb or fingers. Dipping the fingers into warm wax baths and using the wax ball as an exercise tool are beneficial.

Comments

Trapezio-metacarpal joint capsulitis is a common lesion of older females and the results of infiltration are uniformly excellent. Often it is several years before a repeat injection is required, provided the patient does not grossly overuse the joint.

Infiltrating the finger joints can be difficult and sometimes it is necessary to anaesthetize the capsule with some of the solution while trying to enter the joint.

THUMB AND FINGER JOINTS

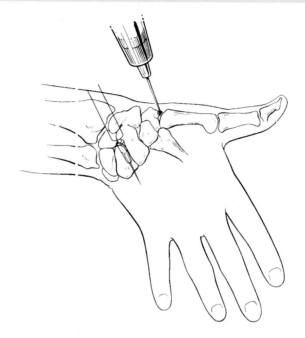

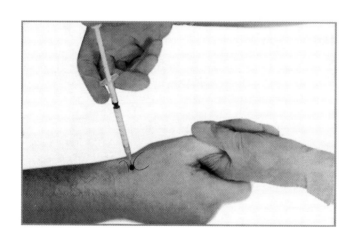

THUMB TENDONS

DE QUERVAIN'S TENOSYNOVITIS

Cause
Overuse of abductor pollicis longus and extensor pollicis brevis

Findings
Pain over base of thumb and over styloid process of radius
Painful: resisted abduction and extension of thumb
            passive flexion of thumb across palm especially with wrist in
            ulnar deviation

Equipment

Syringe	Needle	Kenalog 40	Lidocaine	Total volume
1 ml	25G 0.25″ (0.5 × 16 mm)	10 mg	0.75 ml 2%	1 ml

Anatomy
The abductor pollicis longus and extensor pollicis brevis usually run together in a single sheath on the radial side of the wrist. The styloid process is always tender so comparison should be made with the pain-free side. The two tendons can often be seen when the thumb is held in extension, or can be palpated at the base of the metacarpal.

The aim is to slide the needle between the two tendons and deposit the solution within the sheath.

Technique
- Patient places hand vertically with thumb held in slight flexion
- Identify and mark gap between the two tendons
- Insert needle perpendicularly into gap then slide proximally between the tendons
- Deposit solution as bolus within tendon sheath

Aftercare
Rest for a week with taping of the tendons. This is followed by avoidance of the provoking activity, and a graded strengthening regime

Comments
Provided the wrist is not too swollen, a small sausage-shaped swelling can be seen where the solution distends the tendon sheath.

This is an area where depigmentation or subcutaneous atrophy can occur, especially on thin females. Although recovery can take place, the results may be permanent. The patient should be warned of this possibility.

THUMB TENDONS

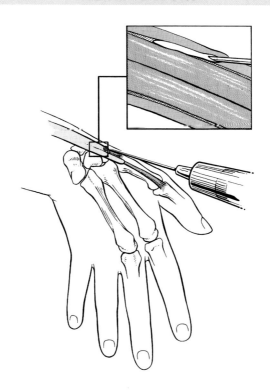

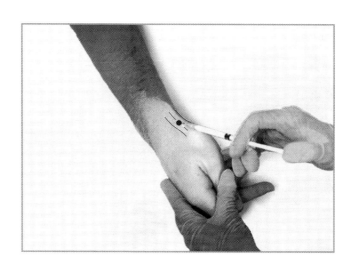

FLEXOR TENDON NODULE

TRIGGER FINGER

Cause

Spontaneous onset – may have osteoarthritis or palpable ganglia in the fingers or hand

Findings

Painful clicking and sometimes locking of finger with inability to extend
A tender nodule can be palpated usually at the base of the finger

Equipment

Syringe	Needle	Kenalog 40	Lidocaine	Total volume
1 ml	25G 0.5" (0.5 × 16 mm)	10 mg	0.75 ml 2%	1 ml

Anatomy

Trigger finger is caused by enlargement of a nodule within the flexor tendon sheath.

Technique

- Patient places hand palm up
- Identify and mark nodule
- Insert needle perpendicularly into nodule and angle distally into sheath
- Deposit solution in a bolus

Aftercare

No particular restriction is placed on the patient's activities.

Comments

This injection is invariably effective. Although the nodule usually remains, it can continue to be asymptomatic indefinitely. Occasionally a slight pop is felt as the needle penetrates the nodule.

FLEXOR TENDON NODULE

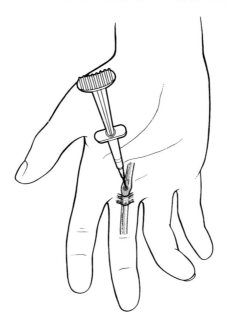

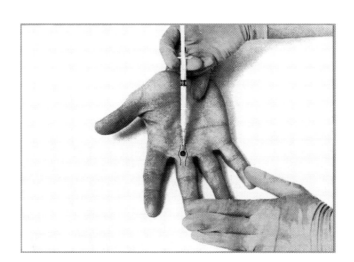

CARPAL TUNNEL

MEDIAN NERVE COMPRESSION UNDER FLEXOR RETINACULUM

Cause
Overuse or trauma
Pregnancy, hypothyroidism, rheumatoid arthritis
Idiopathic

Findings
Pins and needles in the distribution of the median nerve, especially at night.
Pins and needles may be reproduced by tapping the median nerve at the wrist (Tinnel's sign) or by holding the wrist in full flexion for 30 seconds and then releasing (Phalen's sign). Longstanding median nerve compression may show flattening of the thenar eminence.

Equipment

Syringe	Needle	Kenalog 40	Lidocaine	Total volume
1 ml	23G 1.5″ (0.6 × 30 mm)	20 mg		0.5 ml

Anatomy
The flexor retinaculum of the wrist attaches to four sites: the pisiform and the scaphoid, the hook of hamate and the trapezium. It is approximately as wide as the thumb from proximal to distal and the proximal edge lies at the distal wrist crease.

The median nerve lies immediately under the palmaris longus tendon at the mid-point of the wrist, and medial to the flexor carpi radialis tendon. Not every patient will have a palmaris longus so ask the patient to press tip of thumb onto tip of little finger. The crease seen at mid-point of the palm points to the median nerve.

Technique
- Patient places hand palm up
- Identify and mark position of median nerve
- Insert needle at 45° into proximal wrist crease between flexor carpi radialis and nerve. Slide distally until needle point lies under mid-point of retinaculum
- Deposit solution in bolus

Aftercare
The patient rests for a few days and then resumes normal activities. A night splint is often helpful in the early stages after the infiltration and the patient is advised to avoid sleeping with the wrists held in full flexion.

Comments
Care should be taken to avoid inserting the needle too vertically, when it will go into bone, or too horizontally, when it will enter the retinaculum. If the patient experiences pins and needles, the needle is repositioned. Although one injection is often successful, recurrences do occur. Further injections can be given if some relief was obtained, but if the symptoms still recur surgery may be required.

CARPAL TUNNEL

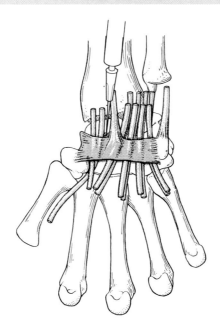

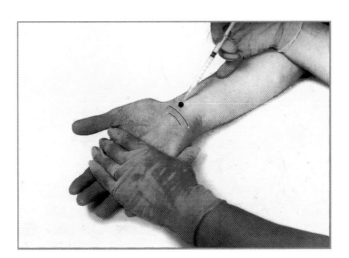

Section 3

Injection techniques: lower limb

HIP JOINT

ACUTE CAPSULITIS

Cause
Osteoarthritis with night pain and severe radiating pain no longer responding to physiotherapy

Findings
Buttock, groin and/or anterior thigh pain
Painful: limitation mostly of passive medial rotation
          less of flexion and abduction
          least of extension
Hard end-feel on passive testing

Equipment

Syringe	Needle	Kenalog 40	Lidocaine	Total volume
5 ml	22G 3–3.5″ (0.7 × 75–90 mm)	40 mg	4 ml 1%	5 ml

Anatomy
The hip joint capsule attaches to the base of the surgical neck of the femur. Therefore, if the needle is inserted to the neck, the solution will be deposited within the capsule. The safest and easiest approach is from the lateral aspect.

The greater trochanter is triangular in shape with a sharp angulation of the apex overhanging the neck. This part is difficult to palpate, especially on patients with excessive adipose tissue, so allow at least a finger's width above the most prominent part of the trochanter for infiltration.

Technique
- Patient lies on pain-free side with lower leg flexed and upper leg straight and resting on pillow so that it lies horizontal
- Identify apex of greater trochanter with finger while passively abducting patient's upper leg
- Insert needle perpendicularly about a finger's width proximal to apex of trochanter until it touches the neck of femur. There is usually no sensation of penetrating the capsule
- Deposit solution in a bolus

Aftercare
Patient gradually increases pain-free activity maintaining range with a home stretching routine, but limits weight-bearing exercise.

Comments
The lateral approach to the hip joint is both simple and safe. It is not necessary to do the technique under fluoroscopy and the procedure is not painful. This injection is usually given to patients who are on a waiting list for surgery. It is successful in giving temporary pain relief and can, if necessary, be repeated at intervals of no less than 3 months. An annual X-ray monitors degenerative change.

HIP JOINT

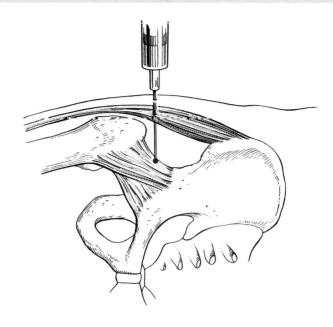

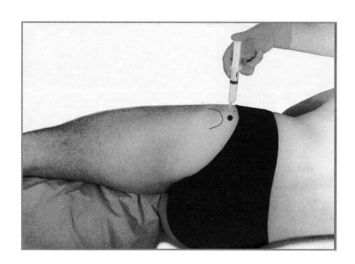

GLUTEAL BURSA

CHRONIC BURSITIS

Cause
Overuse

Findings
Pain and tenderness over the upper lateral quadrant of the buttock
Painful: passive flexion, abduction and adduction
        resisted abduction and extension

Equipment

Syringe	Needle	Kenalog 40	Lidocaine	Total Volume
5 ml	22G 3–3.5″ (0.7 × 75–90 mm)	20 mg	4.5 ml 1%	5 ml

Anatomy
The gluteal bursae are variable in number, size and shape. They can lie deep to the gluteal muscles on the blade of the ilium and also between the layers of the three gluteal muscles. The painful site guides the placement of the needle but comparison between the two sides is essential as this area is always tender.

Technique
- Patient lies on unaffected side with lower leg extended and upper leg flexed
- Identify and mark centre of tender area in upper outer quadrant of buttock
- Insert needle perpendicular to skin until it touches bone of ilium
- Deposit fluid in areas of no resistance while moving needle in a circular manner out towards surface – imagine the needle walking up a spiral staircase

Aftercare
The patient must avoid overusing the leg for a week and can then gradually resume normal activities. Retraining in the causative sporting activity is necessary.

Comments
There are no major blood vessels or nerves in the area of the bursa so the injection is safe. Feeling for a loss of resistance beneath and within the glutei guides the clinician in depositing the fluid.

GLUTEAL BURSA

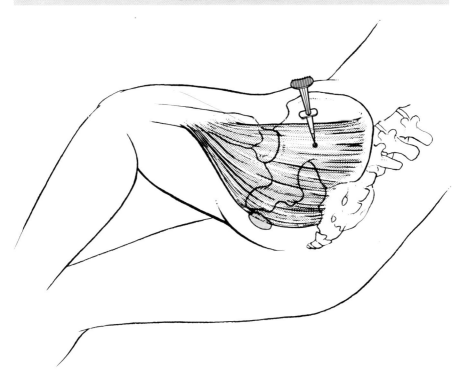

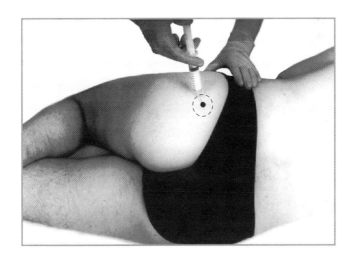

PSOAS BURSA

CHRONIC BURSITIS

Cause
Overuse – especially sports or activities involving repeated hip flexion movements
e.g. hurdling, ballet, javelin throwing, football

Findings
Pain in groin
Painful: passive flexion, adduction, abduction and possibly extension
resisted flexion and adduction
scoop test – semicircular compression of femur from
full flexion to adduction

Equipment

Syringe	Needle	Kenalog 40	Lidocaine	Total volume
5 ml	22G 3–3.5″ (0.7 × 75–90 mm)	20 mg	4.5 ml 1%	5 ml

Anatomy
The psoas bursa lies between the psoas tendon and the anterior aspect of the neck of the femur. It is deep to the three major vessels in the groin – the femoral vein, artery and nerve. For this reason, correct placement of the needle is essential.

Technique
- Patient lies supine
- Identify femoral pulse at mid-point of inguinal ligament. Move three fingers distally and three fingers laterally. The entry point lies in direct line with the anterior superior iliac spine and passes through the medial edge of the sartorius muscle. Mark this spot
- Insert needle at this point and angle 45° cephalad and then 45° medially. Visualize the needle sliding under the three major vessels through the psoas tendon until point touches bone on anterior aspect of neck of femur
- Withdraw slightly and deposit solution in bolus deep to tendon

Aftercare
Absolute avoidance of the activities which irritated the bursa must be maintained for at least a week, then a stretching of hip extension and muscle-balancing programme is initiated.

Comments
Although this injection may appear intimidating to the clinician at the first attempt, the approach outlined above is safe and effective. Very rarely it is possible to catch a lateral branch of the femoral nerve and temporarily anaesthetize the quadriceps. It is best to keep well lateral at the insertion point and if the patient complains of a tingling or burning pain to reposition the needle before depositing solution.

PSOAS BURSA

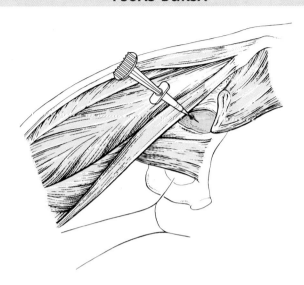

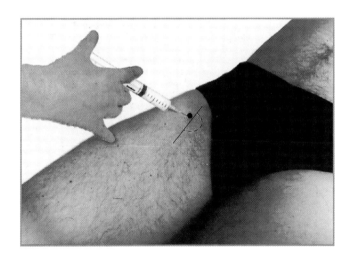

TROCHANTERIC BURSA

ACUTE OR CHRONIC BURSITIS

Cause
Usually a direct blow or fall onto hip
Occasionally overuse or, in the elderly, lying on the same side at night

Findings
Pain and tenderness over greater trochanter
Painful: passive abduction, adduction and possibly flexion and extension of the hip
       resisted abduction

Equipment

Syringe	Needle	Kenalog 40	Lidocaine	Total volume
2 ml	23G 1.25″ (0.6 × 30 mm)	20 mg	1.5 ml 2%	2 ml

Anatomy
The trochanteric bursa lies over the greater trochanter of the femur. It is approximately the size of a golf ball and is usually tender to palpation.

Technique
- Patient lies on unaffected side with lower leg flexed and upper leg extended
- Identify and mark tender area over greater trochanter
- Insert needle at centre of tender area and touch bone of greater trochanter
- Deposit solution by feeling for area of lack of resistance and introducing fluid there

Aftercare
Avoidance of overuse for a week and then gradual return to normal activity. If the cause is lying on a hard mattress, the trochanter can be padded or the mattress changed.

Comments
A fall or direct blow onto the trochanter will often cause a haemorrhagic bursitis. This calls for immediate aspiration of blood prior to the infiltration.

TROCHANTERIC BURSA

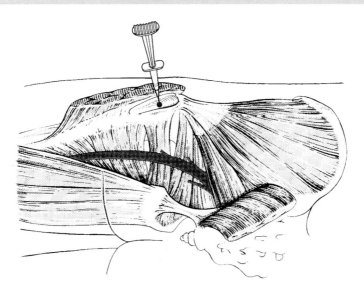

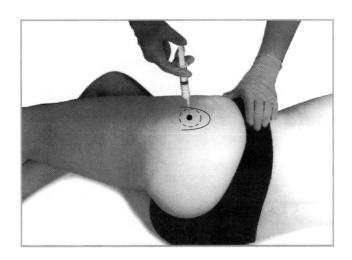

ADDUCTOR TENDONS

CHRONIC TENDINITIS

Cause
Overuse or trauma

Findings
Pain in groin
Painful: resisted adduction
          passive abduction

Equipment

Syringe	Needle	Kenalog 40	Lidocaine	Total volume
2 ml	23G 1.25″ (0.6 × 30 mm)	20 mg	1.5 ml 2%	2 ml

Anatomy
The adductor tendons arise from the pubis and are approximately two fingers wide at their origin. The lesion can lie at the teno-osseous junction or in the body of the tendon. The technique described is for the more common site at the teno-osseous junction.

Technique
- The patient lies supine with leg slightly abducted and laterally rotated
- Identify and mark the origin of the tendon
- Insert needle into tendon angled towards bone of pubis and touch bone
- Pepper solution into teno-osseous junction

Aftercare
Rest for 1 week then graduated stretching and strengthening programme. Deep friction massage may be used to mobilize the scar.

Comments
For the less common site at the body of the tendon, the solution is peppered into the tender area in the body, but deep friction is often more effective here.

ADDUCTOR TENDONS

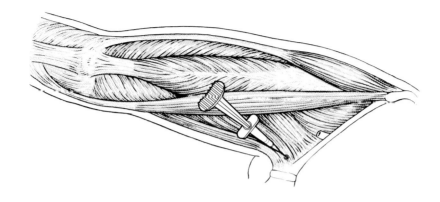

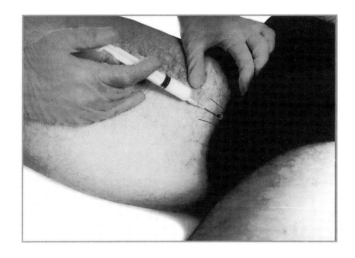

HAMSTRING ORIGIN

CHRONIC TENDINITIS OR ACUTE OR CHRONIC ISCHIAL BURSITIS

Cause
Overuse – such as prolonged riding on horse or bicycle, or running
Trauma – fall onto buttock

Findings
Pain in buttock
Painful: resisted extension
          passive straight leg raise
Very tender over ischial tuberosity

Equipment

Syringe	Needle	Kenalog 40	Lidocaine	Total volume
2 ml	21G 1.5–2″ (0.8 × 40–50 mm)	20 mg	1.5 ml 2%	2 ml

Anatomy
The hamstrings have a common origin arising from the ischial tuberosity. The tendon is approximately three fingers wide here. The ischial bursa lies between the gluteus maximus and the bone of the ischial tuberosity.

Technique
- Patient lies on unaffected side with lower leg straight and upper leg flexed
- Identify ischial tuberosity and mark tendon lying immediately distal
- Insert needle into mid-point of tendon and angle up toward tuberosity to touch bone
- Pepper solution into teno-osseous junction or deposit in bolus into bursa

Aftercare
Avoidance of precipitating activities such as sitting on hard surfaces or prolonged running is maintained for about a week and then graduated stretching and strengthening programme is started.

Comments
Tendinitis and bursitis may occur together at this site, in which case a larger volume is drawn up and both lesions infiltrated. As usual, it is difficult to differentiate between the two lesions, but if there is a history of a fall or friction overuse, and there is extreme tenderness at the tuberosity, bursitis is suspected.

Occasionally, haemorrhagic bursitis can occur as a result of a hard fall. Aspiration of the blood is then performed prior to infiltration.

HAMSTRING ORIGIN

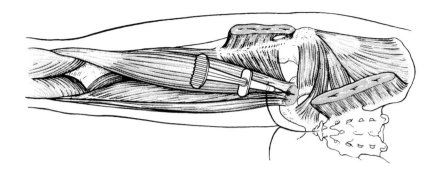

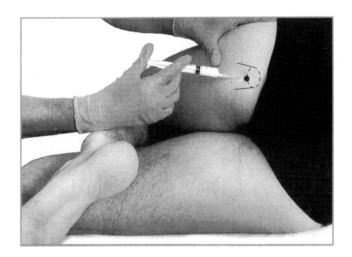

KNEE JOINT

ACUTE OR CHRONIC CAPSULITIS

Cause
Osteoarthritis, rheumatoid arthritis or gout
Trauma

Findings
Pain in knee joint
Painful and limited: more passive flexion than extension with hard end-feel
Possible effusion

Equipment

Syringe	Needle	Kenalog 40	Lidocaine	Total volume
5 ml	21G 1.5–2″ (0.8 × 40–50 mm)	40 mg	4 ml 1%	5 ml

Anatomy
There are several ways to infiltrate or aspirate the knee joint. One way is the lateral approach into the suprapatella pouch just above the lateral pole of the patella; or the medial approach under the medical edge of the patella, as shown here.

Technique
- Patient sits with knee supported
- Identify and mark medial edge of patella
- Insert needle perpendicularly and angle laterally into suprapatella pouch
- Deposit solution as bolus or aspirate if required

Aftercare
The patient avoids undue weight-bearing activity for about a week and then is given strengthening and mobilizing exercises to continue at home.

Comments
The same approach can be used whether infiltrating or aspirating serous fluid or blood.

The injection will give temporary relief from pain and, provided the knee is not overused, this can last for some time. Repeat injections can be given at intervals of not less than 3 months with an annual X-ray to monitor joint degeneration.

KNEE JOINT

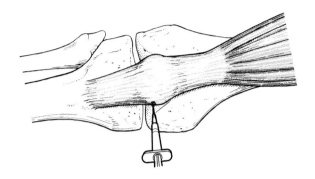

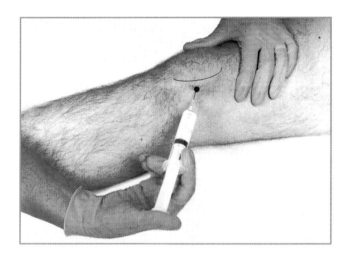

SUPERIOR TIBIO-FIBULAR JOINT

ACUTE OR CHRONIC CAPSULITIS

Cause
Usually trauma such as a fall with forced medial rotation of the foot on a flexed knee

Findings
Pain over joint
Painful: resisted flexion of knee
        full passive medial rotation of knee

Equipment

Syringe	Needle	Kenalog 40	Lidocaine	Total volume
2 ml	23G 1″ (0.6 × 25 mm)	20 mg	1 ml 2%	1.5 ml

Anatomy
The superior tibio-fibular joint line runs medially from superior to inferior. The anterior approach to the joint is safer as the peroneal nerve lies posterior.

Technique
- Patient sits with knee at right angle
- Identify head of fibula and mark joint line medial to it
- Insert needle at mid-point of joint line and aim obliquely laterally to penetrate capsule
- Deposit solution in bolus

Aftercare
Relative rest for about a week and then resumption of normal activities. Strengthening of the biceps femoris may be necessary.

Comments
Occasionally the joint is subluxed and has to be manipulated before infiltration. The condition occasionally occurs after severe ankle sprain.
   The unstable joint can be treated with sclerotherapy.

SUPERIOR TIBIO-FIBULAR JOINT

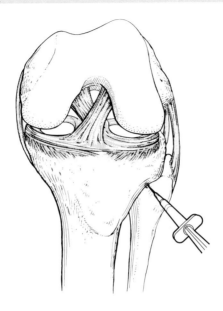

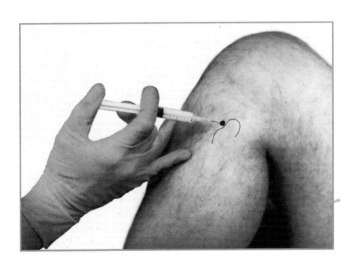

CORONARY LIGAMENT

LIGAMENTOUS SPRAIN

Cause
Trauma – a strong forced rotation of the knee with or without meniscal tear

Findings
Pain usually at medial joint line
Painful: passive lateral rotation
          possibly meniscal tests

Equipment

Syringe	Needle	Kenalog 40	Lidocaine	Total volume
1 ml	25G 0.5″ (0.5 × 16 mm)	10 mg	0.75 ml 2%	1 ml

Anatomy
The coronary ligaments are small thin fibrous bands attaching the menisci to the tibial plateaux.

The medial ligament is more usually affected. It can be found by placing the foot on the table with the knee at right angles and turning the foot into lateral rotation. This brings the tibial plateau into prominence and the tender area is sought by pressing in and down onto the shelf.

Technique
- Patient sits with knee at right angle and planted foot laterally rotated
- Identify and mark tender area on tibial plateau
- Insert needle vertically down onto plateau
- Pepper all along tender area

Aftercare
Early mobilizing exercise to full range of motion without pain is started immediately.

Comments
These ligaments usually respond extremely well to deep friction – it is not uncommon to cure the symptoms in one session. The injection should be kept for where the friction treatment is not available or where the pain is too intense to allow the pressure of the finger.

Tear or subluxation of the meniscus should be treated first by manipulation.

CORONARY LIGAMENT

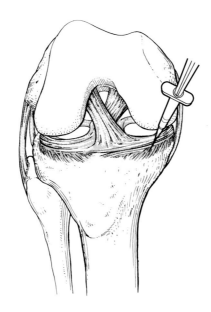

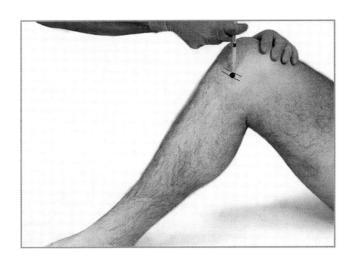

MEDIAL COLLATERAL LIGAMENT

ACUTE OR CHRONIC SPRAIN

Cause
Trauma – typically flexion, valgus and lateral rotation of the knee as in a fall while skiing

Findings
Pain at medial joint line of knee
Painful: passive valgus
           passive lateral rotation of the knee

Equipment

Syringe	Needle	Kenalog 40	Lidocaine	Total volume
2 ml	23G 1.25″ (0.6 × 30 mm)	20 mg	1 ml 2%	1.5 ml

Anatomy
The medial collateral ligament of the knee runs from the medial condyle of the femur to the medial aspect of the shaft of the tibia and is approximately a hand's width long and a good two fingers wide. It is difficult to palpate the ligament as it is so thin and is part of the joint capsule. It is usually sprained at the joint line.

Technique
- Patient lies with knee supported and slightly flexed
- Identify and mark medial joint line and tender area of ligament
- Insert needle at mid-point of tender area. Do not penetrate right through joint capsule
- Pepper solution along width of ligament in two rows

Aftercare
Gentle passive and active movement within the pain-free range is started immediately.

Comments
Sprain of this ligament rarely needs to be injected, as early physiotherapeutic treatment with ice, massage and mobilization is very effective. The injection approach can be used when this treatment is not available or the patient is in a great deal of pain.

MEDIAL COLLATERAL LIGAMENT

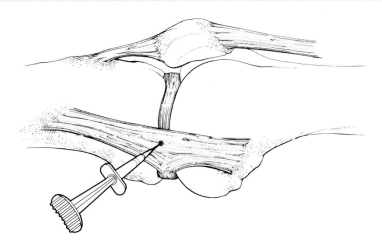

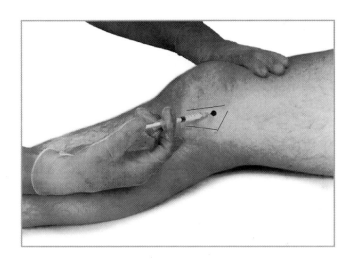

INFRAPATELLA BURSA

ACUTE OR CHRONIC BURSITIS

Cause
Overuse – long distance running or prolonged kneeling
Trauma – direct blow or fall

Findings
Pain anterior knee below patella
Painful: resisted extension of knee
          passive flexion of knee
Tenderness at mid-point of patella tendon

Equipment

Syringe	Needle	Kenalog 40	Lidocaine	Total volume
2 ml	23G 1.25″ (0.6 × 30 mm)	20 mg	1.5 ml 2%	2 ml

Anatomy
There are two infrapatella bursae – one lies superficial and one deep to the tendon. The technique described is for the deep bursa which is more commonly affected.

Technique
• Patient sits with knee supported in slight flexion
• Identify and mark tender area at mid-point of tendon
• Insert needle horizontally beneath tendon from either medial or lateral side. Ensure that the needle does not enter the tendon
• Deposit solution as bolus

Aftercare
The patient must avoid all overuse of the knee for at least a week. Where the cause is occupational, such as in carpet layers, a pad with a hole in it to relieve pressure on the bursa should be used.
   Graded stretching and strengthening exercises are then begun.

Comments
It would be tempting to believe that pain found at mid-point of the patella tendon is caused by tendinitis, but in the experience of the authors this is virtually unknown. Infrapatella tendinitis is found consistently at the proximal teno-osseous junction on the patella, or rarely at insertion into the tibial tubercle. Pain here in an adolescent boy should be considered to be Osgood Schlatter's disease and should not be injected.

INFRAPATELLA BURSA

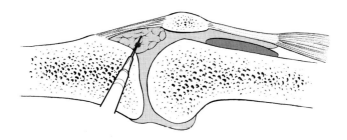

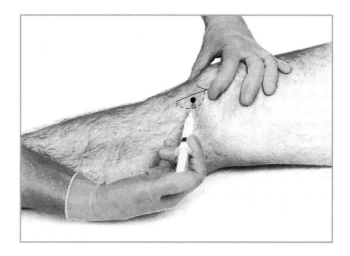

PES ANSEURINE BURSA

CHRONIC BURSITIS

Cause
Overuse – especially dancers or runners

Findings
Pain just proximal to insertion of medial flexors of knee
Painful: resisted flexion of knee

Equipment

Syringe	Needle	Kenalog 40	Lidocaine	Total volume
2 ml	23G 1.25″ (0.6 × 30 mm)	20 mg	1.5 ml 2%	2 ml

Anatomy
The pes anseurine is the combined tendon of insertion of the sartorius, gracilis and semi-tendinosus. It attaches on the medial side of the tibia just below the knee joint line. The bursa lies immediately under the tendon just posterior to its insertion and is extremely tender to palpation in the normal knee.

Technique
- Patient sits with knee supported
- Identify the pes anseurine tendon by making patient strongly flex knee against resistance. Follow the combined tendons distally to where they disappear at insertion into tibia. The bursa is found as an area of extreme tenderness slightly proximal to the insertion. Mark this
- Insert needle into centre of area through tendon until it touches bone
- Deposit solution in bolus

Aftercare
Avoidance of overuse activities for at least a week, when graded stretching and strengthening exercises are started.

Comments
It is important to remember that the bursa is extremely tender to palpation on everybody, so comparison testing must be done on both knees.

PES ANSEURINE BURSA

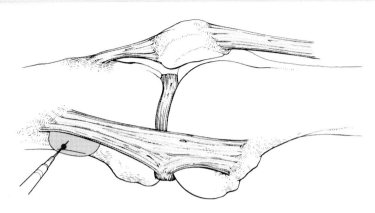

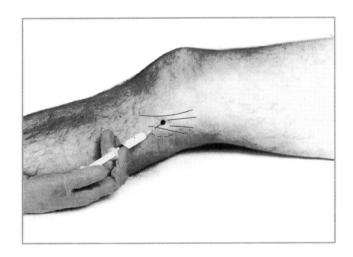

ILIOTIBIAL BAND BURSA

CHRONIC BURSITIS

Cause
Overuse – especially long-distance runners

Findings
Pain on the outer side of the knee above the lateral femoral condyle
Painful: resisted abduction of leg
                passive adduction of leg

Equipment

Syringe	Needle	Kenalog 40	Lidocaine	Total volume
2 ml	23G 1″ (0.6 × 25 mm)	20 mg	1.5 ml 2%	2 ml

Anatomy
The bursa lies deep to the iliotibial band just above the lateral condyle of the femur.

Technique
- Patient sits with knee supported
- Identify and mark tender area on lateral side of femur
- Insert needle into bursa passing through tendon to touch bone
- Deposit solution in bolus

Aftercare
Absolute rest must be maintained for about 10 days and then a stretching and strengthening programme initiated.
   Footwear and running technique must be checked and corrected if necessary.

Comments
The lower end of the iliotibial tract itself can be irritated, but invariably the bursa is also at fault. If both lesions are suspected, infiltration of both at the same time can be performed.

ILIOTIBIAL BAND BURSA

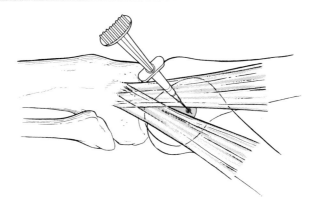

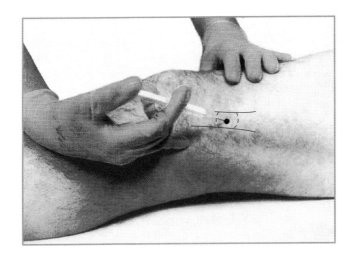

QUADRICEPS EXPANSION

MUSCLE SPRAIN

Cause
Overuse

Findings
Pain usually on superior medial side of patella
Painful: on going down hill or down stairs
                  resisted extension of the knee

Equipment

Syringe	Needle	Kenalog 40	Lidocaine	Total volume
2 ml	25G 0.5″ (0.5 × 16 mm)	10 mg	1.25 ml 2%	2 ml

Anatomy
The quadriceps muscle inserts as an expansion around the borders of the patella. The usual site of the lesion is at the superior medial pole of the patella. This is found by pushing the patella medially with the thumb and palpating up and under the medial edge with a finger to find the tender area.

Technique
• Patient half lies on table with knee relaxed
• Identify and mark tender area usually on medial edge of superior pole of patella
• Insert needle and angle horizontally to touch bone of patella
• Pepper solution along line of insertion

Aftercare
Patient avoids overusing the knee for at least a week and when pain-free begins progressive strengthening and stretching programme.

Comments
This lesion, like the coronary ligament, responds very well to two or three sessions of strong deep friction. The injection is used therefore when the friction is not available, the area is too tender, or to disinflame the expansion prior to friction a week later, in a combination approach. The same technique may be used to inject inflamed plicae around the patella rim.

QUADRICEPS EXPANSION

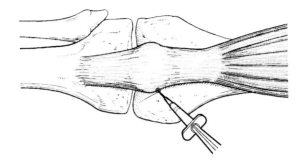

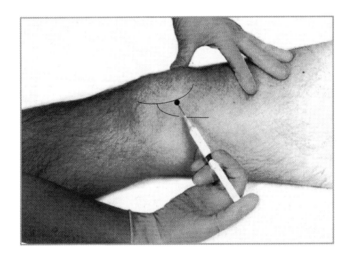

INFRAPATELLA TENDON

CHRONIC TENDINITIS

Cause
Overuse – jumpers and runners

Findings
Pain at inferior pole of patella
Painful: resisted extension of knee

Equipment

Syringe	Needle	Kenalog 40	Lidocaine	Total volume
2 ml	23G 1.25" (0.6 × 30 mm)	20 mg	1.5 ml 2%	2 ml

Anatomy
The infrapatella tendon arises from the inferior pole of the patella and it is here that it is commonly inflamed. The tendon is at least two fingers wide at its origin.

It is an absolute contraindication to inject corticosteroid into the body of the tendon as it is a large, weight-bearing and relatively avascular structure. Tenderness at mid-point of the tendon is usually caused by infrapatella bursitis.

Technique
- Patient sits with knee supported and extended
- Place web of cephalic hand on superior pole of patella and tilt inferior pole up. Identify and mark tender area at origin of tendon on distal end of patella
- Insert needle at mid-point of tendon origin at an angle of 45°
- Pepper solution along tendon in two rows. There should always be some resistance to the needle to ensure that the solution is not being introduced intra-articularly

Aftercare
Absolute rest is recommended for at least 10 days before a stretching and strengthening programme is initiated.

Comments
Injecting the origin of the infrapatella tendon at the inferior pole is very safe, provided adequate rest is maintained afterwards and that no more than two injections are given in one attack.

In the case of the committed athlete, however, alternative treatment such as deep friction, electrotherapy and taping should be considered.

INFRAPATELLA TENDON

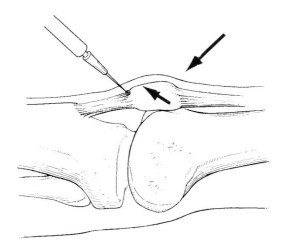

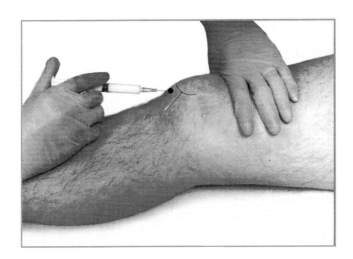

BAKER'S CYST

Cause
Spontaneous insidious onset, usually in osteoarthritic joint

Findings
Obvious swelling in the popliteal fossa – often quite large

Equipment

Syringe	Needle
10 ml	19G 1.5″ (1.1 × 40 mm)

Anatomy
Baker's cyst is a sac of synovial fluid caused by seepage through a defect in the posterior wall of the capsule of the knee joint, or by effusion within the semimembranosus bursa.

The popliteal artery and vein and posterior tibial nerve pass centrally in the popliteal fossa and must be avoided.

Technique
- Patient lies prone
- Mark spot two fingers medial to mid-line of fossa and two fingers below the popliteal crease
- Insert needle at marked spot and angle laterally at 45° angle
- Aspirate at intervals

Aftercare
A firm compression bandage can be applied for a day or two.

Comments
If anything other than clear synovial fluid is removed, a specimen should be sent for culture and the appropriate treatment instigated. Invariably the swelling returns within 6 months to a year but can be re-aspirated if the patient wishes.

BAKER'S CYST

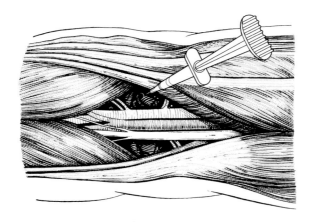

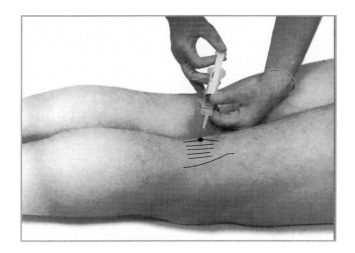

ANKLE JOINT

CHRONIC CAPSULITIS

Cause
Post-trauma – previous fracture or severe injury, often many years later

Findings
Pain at front of, or within, ankle
Painful and limited: more passive plantarflexion
less passive dorsiflexion

Equipment

Syringe	Needle	Kenalog 40	Lidocaine	Total volume
2 ml	23G 1.25" (0.6 × 30 mm)	30 mg	1.25 ml 2%	2 ml

Anatomy
The easiest and safest entry point to the ankle joint is at the junction of the tibia and fibula just above the talus. A small triangular space can be palpated there.

Technique
- Patient lies with foot slightly plantarflexed
- Identify and mark small triangular space by passively flexing and extending the ankle while palpating
- Insert needle into joint angling slightly medially to pass through capsule
- Deposit solution as bolus

Aftercare
Avoidance of excessive weight-bearing activities is maintained for at least a week. The patient should be warned that heavy overuse of the foot will cause a recurrence of symptoms and therefore long-distance running should be avoided. Weight control is also advised.

Comments
The ankle joint rarely causes problems except after severe trauma or fracture, and then often many years later. The infiltration is usually very successful in giving long-lasting pain relief and can be repeated if necessary at intervals of at least 3 months with an annual X-ray to monitor degenerative changes.

ANKLE JOINT

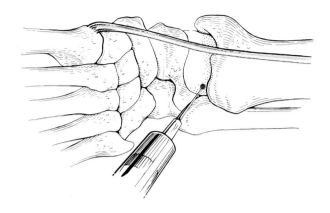

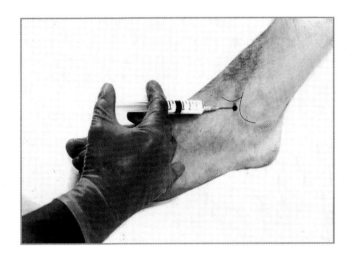

SUBTALAR JOINT

CHRONIC CAPSULITIS

Cause
Trauma – usually after fracture or severe impaction injury, often many years later
Obesity

Findings
Pain deep in medial and lateral sides of heel
Painful and limited: passive adduction of the calcaneus

Equipment

Syringe	Needle	Kenalog 40	Lidocaine	Total volume
2 ml	23G 1.25″ (0.6 × 30 mm)	30 mg	1.25 ml 2%	2 ml

Anatomy
The subtalar joint is divided by an oblique septum into anterior and posterior portions. It is slightly easier to enter the joint just above the sustentaculum tali which is a bump of bone lying a thumb's width below the medial malleolus.

Technique
- Patient lies on side with foot supported so that medial aspect of heel faces upwards
- Identify bump of sustentaculum tali
- Insert needle perpendicularly immediately above and slightly posterior to sustentaculum tali
- Deposit half solution here
- Withdraw needle slightly and angle obliquely anteriorly through septum into anterior compartment of joint space and deposit remaining solution here

Aftercare
Avoidance of excessive weight-bearing activities for at least a week.
Orthotics and weight control are helpful in preventing recurrence

Comments
This is a difficult injection to perform due to the anatomical shape of the joint. It can be repeated at infrequent intervals if necessary.

SUBTALAR JOINT

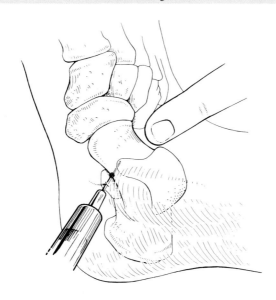

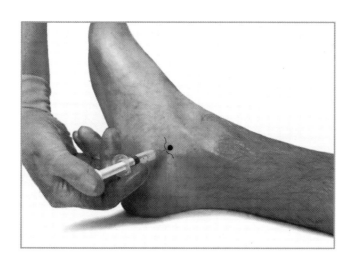

DELTOID LIGAMENT

ACUTE OR CHRONIC SPRAIN

Cause
Trauma
Obesity
Overpronation of the foot

Findings
Pain over medial side of heel below medial malleolus
Painful: passive eversion of ankle in plantarflexion

Equipment

Syringe	Needle	Kenalog 40	Lidocaine	Total volume
1 ml	25G 0.5″ (0.5 × 16 mm)	10 mg	0.75 ml 2%	1 ml

Anatomy
The deltoid ligament is a strong triangular structure with two layers. It runs from the medial malleolus to the sustentaculum tali on the calcaneum and to the tubercle on the navicular. Sprains here are not as common as at the lateral ligament, but because they do not seem to respond well to friction and mobilization, injection is worth trying. The inflamed part is usually at the origin on the malleolus.

Technique
- Patient sits with medial side of foot accessible
- Identify lower border of medial malleolus and mark mid-point of ligament
- Insert needle and angle upwards to touch bone at mid-point of ligament
- Pepper solution along attachment to bone

Aftercare
To prevent recurrence, the biomechanics of the foot must be carefully checked. Almost always an orthotic is necessary and, in the overweight patient, advice on diet must be given

Comments
An uncommon but universally successful injection.

DELTOID LIGAMENT

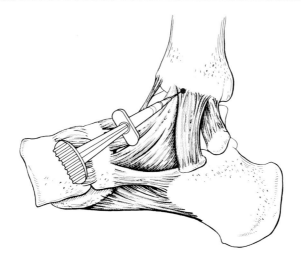

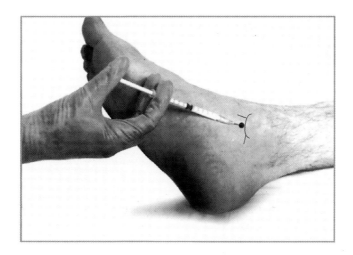

LATERAL LIGAMENT

ACUTE LIGAMENTOUS SPRAIN

Cause
Inversion injury

Findings
Pain at lateral side of ankle
Painful: passive inversion of ankle

Equipment

Syringe	Needle	Kenalog 40	Lidocaine	Total volume
1 ml	25G 0.5" (0.5 × 16 mm)	10 mg	0.75 ml 2%	1 ml

Anatomy
The anterior talo-fibular ligament runs medially from the anterior inferior edge of the lateral malleolus to attach to the talus. It is a thin structure and is approximately the width of the little finger.

The bifurcate calcaneo-cuboid ligament runs from the calcaneus to the cuboid and is often also involved in ankle sprains. Both ligaments run parallel to the sole of the foot.

Technique
- Patient lies supported on table
- Identify and mark anterior inferior edge of lateral malleolus
- Insert needle to touch bone
- Pepper half solution around origin of ligament
- Turn needle and pepper remainder into insertion on talus

Aftercare
Patient keeps ankle moving within pain-free range. For the first few days ice, elevation and taping in eversion are helpful

Comments
This lesion responds very well in the acute stage to a regime of ice, elevation, gentle massage, active and passive mobilization and taping. The injection can be used where this treatment is not available, where the pain is very acute or where conservative treatment has failed in the chronic stage.

LATERAL LIGAMENT

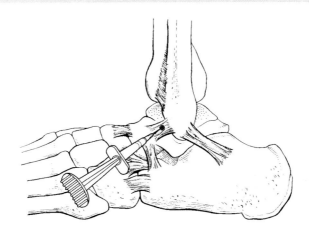

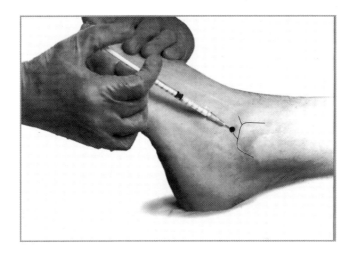

ACHILLES TENDON

CHRONIC TENDINITIS

Cause
Overuse

Findings
Pain at posterior aspect of ankle
Painful: resisted plantarflexion on one foot or from full dorsiflexion

Equipment

Syringe	Needle	Kenalog 40	Lidocaine	Total volume
2 ml	23G 1.25″ (0.6 × 30 mm)	20 mg	1.5 ml 2%	2 ml

Anatomy
The achilles tendon lies at the end of the gastrocnemius as it inserts into the posterior surface of the calcaneus. It is absolutely contraindicated to infiltrate into the *body* of the tendon as it is a large, weight-bearing, relatively avascular tendon with a known propensity to rupture.

Technique
- Patient lies prone with foot held in dorsiflexion over end of bed. This keeps the tendon under tension and facilitates the procedure
- Identify and mark tender area of tendon – usually along the sides
- Insert needle on medial side and angle parallel to tendon. Slide needle along side of tendon, taking care not to enter into tendon itself
- Deposit half solution while slowly withdrawing needle
- Insert needle on lateral side and repeat procedure with remaining half of solution

Aftercare
Absolute avoidance of any overuse is essential for about 10 days. Deep friction to the site should then be given a few times, even if the patient is asymptomatic, to prevent recurrence. When pain-free, graded stretching and strengthening exercises are begun and should be continued indefinitely. Orthotics and retraining in the causal activity are often necessary.

Comments
Although there are reports of tendon rupture after injection here, this has usually occurred as a result of repeated injections of large dose and volume into the body of the tendon and with excessive exercise post-injection. However, it is advisable to scan the tendon prior to injecting to ascertain the extent of the degeneration. Depositing the solution along the sides is safe and effective but should not be repeated more than once in one attack. The committed athlete may prefer to receive deep friction and a graduated stretching/strenghtening programme.

ACHILLES TENDON

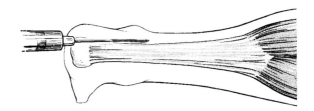

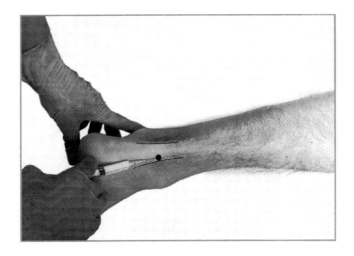

ACHILLES BURSA

CHRONIC BURSITIS

Cause
Overuse – runners and dancers

Findings
Pain posterior to tibia and anterior to body of achilles tendon
Painful: resisted plantarflexion especially at end range
full passive plantarflexion

Equipment

Syringe	Needle	Kenalog 40	Lidocaine	Total volume
2 ml	23G 1.25″ (0.6 × 30 mm)	20 mg	1.5 ml 2%	2 ml

Anatomy
The achilles bursa lies in the triangular space anterior to the tendon and posterior to the base of the tibia and the upper part of the calcaneus.

It is important to differentiate between tendinitis and bursitis here as both are caused by overuse. In bursitis there is usually more pain on full passive plantarflexion when the heel is pressed up against the back of the tibia, thereby squeezing the bursa. Also, palpation of the bursa is very sensitive and the pain is usually felt more at the end of rising on tip-toe rather than during the movement.

Technique
- Patient lies prone with foot held in some dorsiflexion
- Identify and mark tender area
- Insert needle into bursa from the lateral aspect avoiding piercing the tendon
- Deposit solution as bolus

Aftercare
Avoid overuse activities for at least a week then start a stretching programme. Dancers need to be careful not to over-point.

Comments
The important part of this injection is to avoid penetrating the achilles tendon and depositing the solution there. Any resistance to the needle requires immediate withdrawal and repositioning well anterior to the tendon.

ACHILLES BURSA

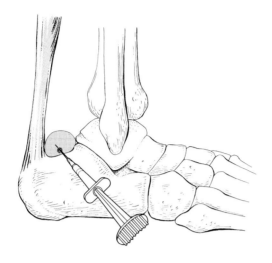

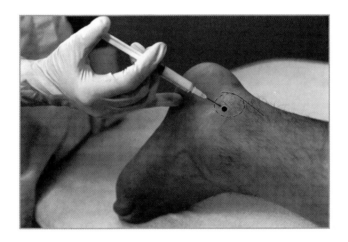

MIDTARSAL JOINTS

ACUTE OR CHRONIC CAPSULITIS

Cause
Overuse or trauma – female ballet dancers who over-point or football players

Findings
Pain on dorsum of foot – usually at third metatarso-cuneiform joint line
Painful and limited: adduction and inversion of midtarsal joints

Equipment

Syringe	Needle	Kenalog 40	Lidocaine	Total volume
2 ml	23G 1″ (0.6 × 25 mm)	20 mg	1.5 ml 2%	1.5 ml

Anatomy
There are several joints in the mid-tarsus, each with its own capsule. Gross passive testing followed by local joint gliding and palpation should identify the joint involved.

Technique
- Patient lies with foot supported in neutral
- Identify and mark tender joint line
- Insert needle down into joint space
- Pepper some solution into capsule and remainder as bolus into joint cavity

Aftercare
Avoidance of excessive weight-bearing activities for at least a week.
   Mobilizing and strengthening exercises and retraining of causal activities follow. Orthotics and weight control, if necessary, are useful additions.

Comments
This is a universally successful treatment provided sensible attention is paid to after-care.

MIDTARSAL JOINTS

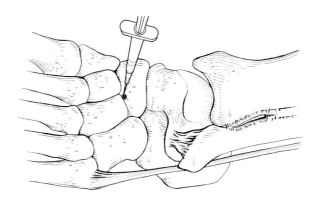

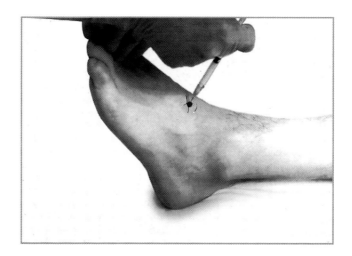

TOE JOINTS

ACUTE OR CHRONIC CAPSULITIS

Cause
Overuse or trauma
Hallux valgus

Findings
Pain in toe joint
Painful and limited: extension of the big toe, flexion of other toes

Equipment

Syringe	Needle	Kenalog 40	Lidocaine	Total volume
2 ml	25G 0.5″ (0.5 × 16 mm)	20 mg	1 ml 2%	1.5 ml

Anatomy
The first metatarso-phalangeal joint line is found by palpating the space produced at the base of the metacarpal on the dorsal aspect, while passively flexing and extending the toe.

Technique
- Patient lies with foot supported
- Identify and mark joint line and distract big toe with one hand
- Insert needle perpendicularly into joint space avoiding extensor hallucis tendon
- Deposit solution as bolus

Aftercare
Avoidance of excessive weight-bearing activities for at least a week, together with taping of the joint and a toe pad between the toes.

Comments
As with the thumb joint injection, this treatment can be very long-lasting.

The other toe joints are injected from the medial or lateral aspect while under traction.

TOE JOINTS

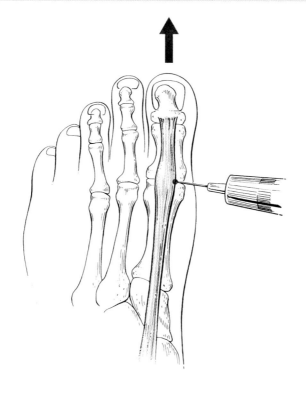

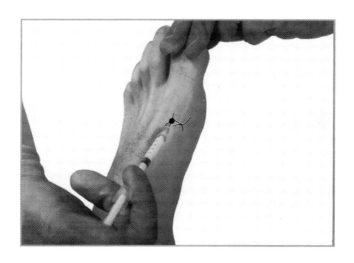

PERONEAL TENDONS

ACUTE OR CHRONIC TENDINITIS

Cause
Overuse

Findings
Pain at lateral side of ankle or foot
Painful: resisted eversion of the foot
Tender area above, behind or below the lateral malleolus

Equipment

Syringe	Needle	Kenalog 40	Lidocaine	Total volume
1 ml	25G 0.5" (0.5 × 16 mm)	10 mg	0.75 ml 2%	1 ml

Anatomy
The peroneus longus and brevis run together in a synovial sheath behind the lateral malleolus. The longus then divides to pass under the arch of the foot and brevis inserts into the base of the fifth metatarsal.

The division of the two tendons is the entry point for the needle and can be found by having the patient hold the foot in strong eversion and palpating for the V-shaped fork of the tendons.

Technique
- Patient lies supine with foot supported in some medial rotation
- Identify and mark division of the two tendons
- Insert needle perpendicularly at this point, turn and slide horizontally under skin towards malleolus
- Deposit solution into combined tendon sheath. There should be minimal resistance and often a sausage-shaped bulge is observed

Aftercare
Avoidance of any overuse for about a week. Resolution of symptoms should then lead to consideration of change in footwear, orthotics and strengthening of the evertors.

Comments
Occasionally the tendinitis occurs at the insertion of the peroneus brevis. The same amount of solution is then peppered into the teno-osseous junction by inserting the needle parallel to the skin to touch the base of the fifth metatarsal.

PERONEAL TENDONS

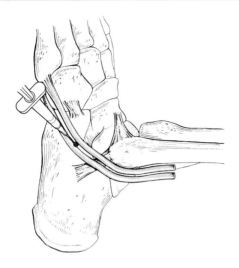

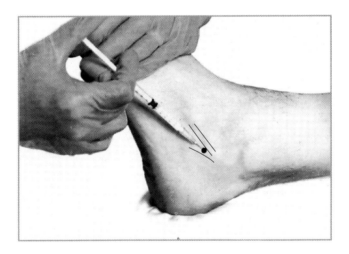

PLANTAR FASCIA

ACUTE FASCIITIS

Cause
Idiopathic, overuse, poor footwear

Findings
Pain on medial aspect of heel pad on putting foot to ground in the morning
Tender area over medial edge of origin of fascia from calcaneus

Equipment

Syringe	Needle	Kenalog 40	Lidocaine	Total volume
2 ml	21G 1.5–2″ (0.8 × 40–50 mm)	20 mg	1.5 ml 2%	2 ml

Anatomy
The plantar fascia, or long plantar ligament, arises from the medial and lateral tubercles on the inferior surface of the calcaneus. The lesion is always found at the medial head and the area of irritation can easily be palpated by deep pressure with the thumb.

Technique
- Patient lies prone with foot supported in dorsiflexion
- Identify tender area on heel
- Insert needle perpendicularly into medial side of soft part of sole just distal to heel pad. Advance at 45° towards calcaneus until it touches bone
- Pepper solution in two rows into fascia at its medial bony origin

Aftercare
A heel support is used for at least a week after the injection, followed by intrinsic muscle exercise and stretching of the fascia. Standing on a golf ball to apply deep friction can be helpful and orthotics can be applied. Taping can also be used.

Comments
Although this would appear to be an extremely painful injection, this approach is much kinder than inserting the needle straight through the heel pad, and patients tolerate it well.

PLANTAR FASCIA

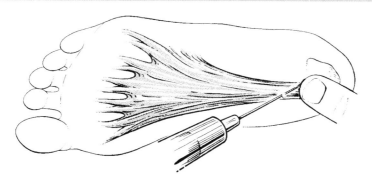

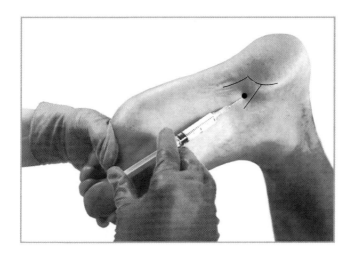

Section 4

Advanced techniques

SPINAL INJECTIONS

There is some controversy in the literature regarding spinal injections[98,99, 127–134]. Depot steroids are not licensed for spinal use[135,136], but rheumatologists, pain specialists and others use these injections extensively.

Corticosteroids, often mixed with a local anaesthetic, are injected into the epidural space (via the caudal or lumbar route) and around nerve roots for the relief of back pain or sciatica, into or around facet joints for the relief of back and referred limb pain, and into muscle trigger points. Performing the injection under fluoroscopy can ensure correct placement of spinal injections[137,139], but many doctors perform these techniques 'blind' and obtain satisfactory results.

Blind caudal epidural injections are correctly placed in only two out of three attempts, even when the operator is confident of accurate placement. When the operator is less certain, the success rate is less than half. If the patient is obese the success rate reduces even further[137]. In the past, large volumes have been injected into the epidural space[138], however, a total injection volume of 8 ml is sufficient for a caudal epidural injection to reach the L4/5 level[139].

The number needed to treat (NNT) with epidural corticosteroids for greater than 75% pain relief in the short term (1–60 days) is 7 (confidence interval = 5–16). The NNT for greater than 50% pain relief in the long term (3–12 months) is 13 (CI = 7–314)[99].

Selective nerve-root injections of corticosteroids (under X-ray control) are significantly more effective than those of bupivacaine alone in obviating the need for operative decompression for 13–28 months following the injections in operative candidates. This finding suggests that patients who have lumbar radicular pain at one or two levels should be considered for treatment with selective nerve-root injections of corticosteroids prior to operative intervention[132].

Sclerosant injections are used to treat back pain with ligamentous insufficiency[140]. They are ineffective in patients with very long-standing (e.g. 10 years) back pain and features of psychosocial distress[141], and are not shown here.

A Cochrane systematic review recommends that because of the tendency towards positive results favouring injection therapy and the minor side-effects reported by the reviewed studies, there is at the moment no justification for abandoning injection therapy in patients with low back pain. However, because of the lack of statistically significant results, as well as the lack of well-designed trials, a solid foundation for the effectiveness of injection therapy is also lacking[133].

Safety precautions and strict aseptic techniques are the same as for all injections but an additional hazard is the rare possibility of an intrathecal injection of local anaesthetic. For this reason, we recommend the use of corticosteroid alone, without the addition of local anaesthetic. The benefit of the brief relief of pain and the diagnostic information thereby obtained does not outweigh the potential risks. Normal saline can be added if additional volume is required.

For physicians using this guide, there follows a description of a few spinal injections which can be safely carried out in an outpatient setting provided resuscitation facilities are available and the simple guidelines suggested are strictly followed. We strongly recommend, however, that doctors attend recognized training courses and undergo a period of supervised practice with an experienced colleague before attempting them on their own. These injections are not intended to be given by physiotherapists.

CERVICAL FACET JOINT

ACUTE OR CHRONIC CAPSULITIS

Causes
Osteoarthritis
Trauma

Findings
Pain in posterior neck, up to head, into scapular or to point of shoulder
Increased by sleeping in awkward positions and end-of-range movement
Painful and/or limited: rotation, side flexion and extension
Tender over one or more facet joints

Equipment

Syringe	Needle	Kenalog 40	Total volume
1 ml	23G 1.25–2″ (0.6 × 30–50 mm)	20 mg	0.5 ml

Anatomy
The facet or zygaphophyseal joints in the cervical spine are plane joints lying at angles of approximately 30–45° to the vertical. They can be palpated by identifying the spinous process and moving two fingers' width laterally. The affected levels are sensitive to pressure.

Technique
- Patient lies on unaffected side with roll under neck. The neck is held in flexion and slight side flexion away from the painful side
- Identify and mark the tender joint
- Insert needle just distal to joint parallel to the spinous processes at an angle of 45° cephalad. Pass through the thick extensors aiming towards patient's upper ear until point touches bone. Ensure needle remains parallel to spinous process at all times and does not pass medially
- Gently 'walk' along bone until needle passes into joint capsule
- Deposit solution in bolus intracapsular or pepper pericapsular

Aftercare
Patient maintains gentle movement, continues correct posture and is careful to sleep with the correct number of pillows to maintain the head in a neutral position.

Comments
We strongly recommend that this technique is practised first with an experienced clinician.

Although this appears to be an alarming injection, it is perfectly safe provided great care is taken that the needle always lies parallel to the spinous process and never at any time angles medially. The results in the osteoarthritic neck can be good for several months or even years, provided the patient does not strain the neck and maintains mobility and good posture.

CERVICAL FACET JOINT

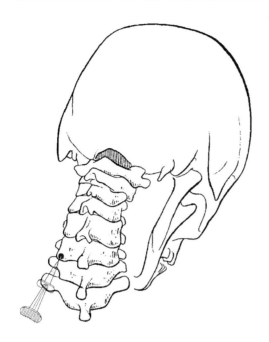

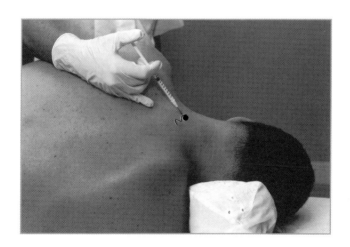

LUMBAR FACET JOINT

CHRONIC CAPSULITIS

Cause
Osteoarthritis or traumatic capsulitis
Spondylolysis/spondylolysthesis
Ankylosing spondylitis

Findings
Unilateral low back pain, sometimes with dull vague aching down leg
Painful and or/limited: extension, both side flexions and less flexion of lumbar spine
In younger patients with spondylolysis, usually most painful movement is combined extension with side flexion to the painful side

Equipment

Syringe	Needle	Kenalog 40	Total volume
1 ml	22G 3–3.5″ (0.7 × 75–90 mm)	40 mg	1 ml

Anatomy
The lower lumbar facet or zygaphophyseal joints lie lateral to the spinous processes – approximately one finger width at L3, one and a half at L4 and two fingers' width at L5. They cannot be palpated but are located by marking a vertical line along the centre of the spinous processes and horizontal lines across *between* each process. The posterior capsule of the joint is found by inserting the needle the correct distance for that level laterally on the horizontal line.

Technique
- Patient lies prone on small pillow to aid localization of the spinous interspace
- Identify and mark levels for infiltration
- Insert needle at first selected level vertically down to capsule. If the capsule is not found immediately, gently 'walk' needle around bone until a ligamentous end-point is reached
- Deposit solution into and around capsule
- Withdraw needle and repeat at different levels if necessary

Aftercare
Avoidance of excessive movement while maintaining comfortable activity. Abdominal strengthening exercises should be performed regularly.

Comments
We strongly recommend that this technique is practised first with an experienced clinician.

Some practitioners recommend injection of the lumbar facets under fluoroscopy, but they can be safely reached in the above manner provided one feels for the end-point of the needle on bone.

LUMBAR FACET JOINT

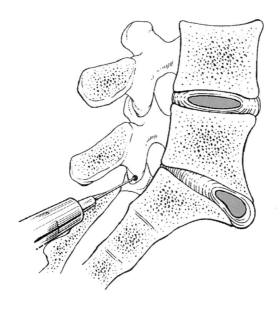

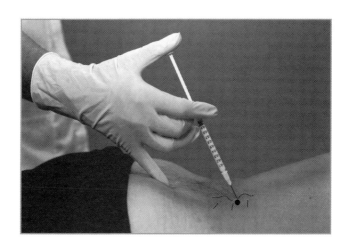

LUMBAR NERVE ROOT

NERVE ROOT INFLAMMATION

Cause
Spinal stenosis
Nerve-root entrapment

Findings
Acute or chronic severe sciatica with or without root signs
Painful: flexion and side bending usually away from painful side
straight leg raise, foot dorsiflexion and neck flexion, slump test

Equipment

Syringe	Needle	Kenalog 40	Total volume
1 ml	22G 3–3.5″ (0.7 × 75–90 mm)	40 mg	1 ml

Anatomy
The lumbar nerve roots emerge obliquely from the vertebral canals between the transverse processes at the level of the spinous process. Draw a vertical line along the centre of the spinous processes and horizontal lines at each spinous level. Two fingers' width laterally along the horizontal line marks entry site for the needle.

Technique
- Patient lies prone over small pillow to aid localization of spinous processes
- Identify spinous process of level required and mark spot along horizontal line
- Insert needle two fingers lateral to spinous process. Pass needle perpendicularly to depth of about 2.5–3 inches (6–7 cm)
- Aspirate to ensure needle is not intrathecal
- Deposit solution in bolus

Aftercare
Patient keeps mobile within pain limits and is reassessed 1 week later. Repeat as necessary.

Comments
We strongly recommend that this technique is practised first with an experienced clinician.

This injection is especially effective when the patient is in severe pain and conservative manual therapy techniques are impossible. It can also be given when caudal epidural has proved unsuccessful – the caudal is technically an easier procedure. The needle must be repositioned if it encounters bone at a distance of about 2″ (5 cm) (lamina or facet joint) or if the patient complains of sharp 'electric shock' (nerve root). If clear fluid is aspirated the needle is intrathecal and the procedure must be abandoned and attempted a few days later. More than one level can be infiltrated at a time.

LUMBAR NERVE ROOT

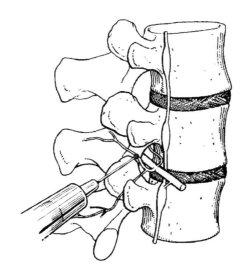

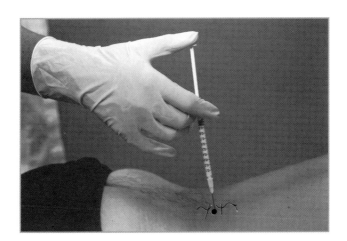

SACRO-ILIAC JOINT

ACUTE OR CHRONIC STRAIN OR CAPSULITIS

Cause
Acute sacro-iliitis
Chronic ligamentous pain after successful manipulation
Ankylosing spondylitis

Findings
Usually female – often pre- or post-partum
Trauma
Pain after rest, long periods of sitting or standing
Pain over buttock, groin or occasionally down posterior thigh to calf
Pain on stressing: posterior ligaments in hip flexion, adduction in flexion and transversely; anterior ligaments in 4 test (combined lateral rotation and abduction)

Equipment

Syringe	Needle	Kenalog 40	Lidocaine	Total volume
2 ml	21G 1.5–2″ (0.8 × 40–50 mm)	20 mg	1.5 ml 20%	2 ml

Anatomy
The joint is angled obliquely postero-anteriorly with the angle being more acute in the female. The dimples at the top of the buttocks indicate the position of the posterior superior iliac spines. The easiest entry point is usually found just below and slightly medial to the spines.

Technique
- Patient lies prone over small pillow
- Identify and mark posterior superior iliac spine on affected side
- Insert needle a thumb's width medial to this bony landmark or dimple at level of second sacral spinous process and angle obliquely lateral at an angle of 45°
- Pass needle between sacrum and ilium until a ligamentous resistance is felt
- Deposit solution in bolus within joint if possible, or pepper posterior capsule

Aftercare
Movement within the pain-free range is encouraged – a lunging motion with the foot up on a chair can help relieve pain. A temporary belt is worn if the joint is unstable and sclerosing injections can be used to increase stability.

Comments
The needle often comes up against bone when attempting this injection and then has to be manoeuvred around to allow for the variations in bony shape before entering the joint space.

It is unusual to have to repeat this injection and the joint can often be successfully manipulated if necessary a week later.

SACRO-ILIAC JOINT

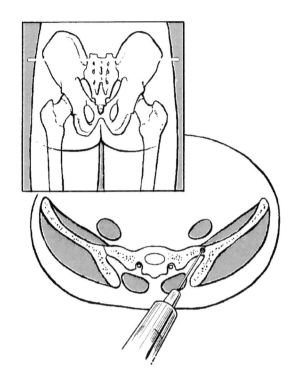

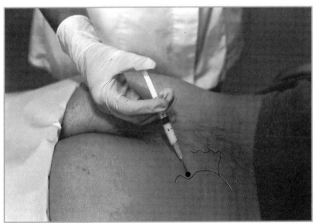

COCCYX

STRAIN OF COCCYGEAL LIGAMENTS

Cause
Trauma
Prolonged sitting on hard surfaces

Findings
Pain over coccyx

Equipment

Syringe	Needle	Kenalog 40	Lidocaine	Total volume
1 ml	23G 1″ (0.6 × 25 mm)	10 mg	0.75 ml 2%	1 ml

Anatomy
The coccygeal ligaments are palpated on the dorsal and ventral surfaces. The bone may be found to be hyperflexed or even twisted.

Technique
- Patient lies prone over small pillow
- Identify and mark tender site on dorsum of coccyx
- Insert needle down to touch bone
- Pepper around into tender ligaments

Aftercare
Advise patient to avoid sitting on hard surfaces and to use a ring cushion. At follow-up 1 week later mobilization or manipulation of the coccyx can be used.

Comments
Pain in this area can be symptomatic of psychological or psychosexual distress, in which case the appropriate referral is required. With somatic pain the protocol above appears to work either extremely well or not at all. Surgery is not usually indicated.

COCCYX

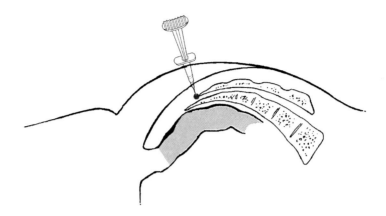

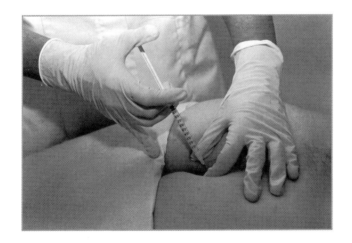

CAUDAL EPIDURAL

ACUTE OR CHRONIC LOW BACK PAIN OR SCIATICA

Cause
Disc lesion
Acute nerve entrapment

Findings
Central or bilateral pain in low back with or without sciatica or root signs
Usually painful flexion and side flexion away from painful side and nerve root tension signs

Equipment

Syringe	Needle	Kenalog 40	Total volume
1 ml	21G 1.5–2″ (0.8 × 40–50 mm)	40 mg	1 ml

Anatomy
The spinal cord ends at the level of L1 and the thecal sac at S2 in most individuals. The aim of this injection is to pass a disinflaming solution through the sacral hiatus and up the canal so that it bathes the inflamed disc, dura mater and nerve roots centrally. The sacral cornua are two prominences that can be palpated at the apex of an equilateral triangle drawn from the posterior superior spines on the ileum to the coccyx. There is a thick ligament at the entrance to the canal. The angle of the curve of the canal varies widely.

Technique
- Patient lies prone over small pillow
- Identify sacral cornua with thumb
- Insert needle horizontally between cornua and pass through ligament
- Pass needle slightly up canal adjusting angle to curve of sacrum
- Aspirate to ensure needle has not penetrated thecal sac or blood vessel
- Slowly inject solution into extradural space while talking to patient
- Keep hand on sacrum to palpate for swelling caused by supra-sacral injection

Aftercare
The patient can continue to do whatever is comfortable and is seen a week later. If the injection has helped it can be repeated at 1- or 2-week intervals as long as improvement continues.

Comments
We recommend that this technique is practised first with an experienced clinician.
  Caudal epidural is safe and effective provided[137]:
- there is no allergy to local anaesthetic (not used in this method)
- no local sepsis
- patient is not on anticoagulant therapy.

We recommend that in the outpatient setting no local anaesthetic is used.

CAUDAL EPIDURAL

Occasionally the canal is difficult to enter – this may be because of a bifid or very small canal or because the angle of the canal is very concave. Removal of the needle and re-angulation may be necessary.

If clear fluid or blood is aspirated at any point the procedure is abandoned and attempted a few days later. If the patient feels faint or dizzy during the injection, stop injecting and wait for the symptoms to go. If they do not, abandon the procedure.

Temporary reproduction of the patient's pain during the infiltration is a good sign that the treatment will be successful.

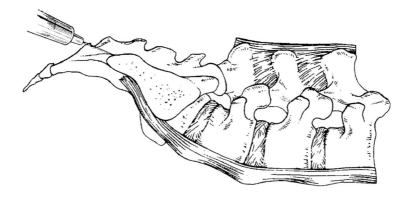

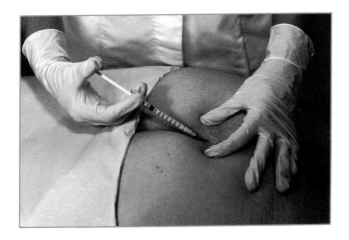

TEMPORO-MANDIBULAR JOINT

ACUTE OR CHRONIC CAPSULITIS

Cause
Trauma – often after a car accident
Osteoarthritis
Meniscal tear

Findings
Headaches
Pain over joint
Painful: on opening, deviation or protrusion of jaw with asymmetry of movement
clicking or locking

Equipment

Syringe	Needle	Kenalog 40	Lidocaine	Total volume
1 ml	25G 0.5" (0.5 × 16 mm)	10 mg	0.75 ml 2%	1 ml

Anatomy
The temporomandibular joint space can be palpated just in front of the ear while the patient opens and closes the mouth. A meniscus lies within the joint and the needle must be placed below this in order to enter the joint space. The joint can be infiltrated most easily when the jaw is held wide open.

Technique
- Patient lies on unaffected side with head supported and mouth held open
- Identify and mark joint space
- Insert needle vertically into inferior compartment of joint space below meniscus. It may be necessary to manoeuvre needle about to avoid meniscus
- Deposit solution in bolus

Aftercare
The patient should avoid excessive movement of the jaw such as biting on a large apple or hard food. Gentle active movements and isometric exercises are carried out. A guard to prevent grinding the teeth at night and/or the advice of an orthodontist may be necessary.

Comments
If the meniscus is displaced, reduction must be attempted before giving the injection.

TEMPORO-MANDIBULAR JOINT

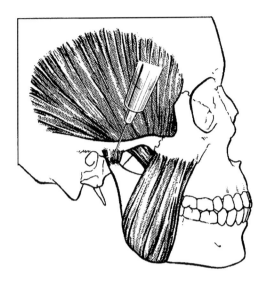

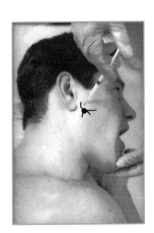

APPENDIX 1

PERIPHERAL JOINT AND SOFT-TISSUE INJECTIONS

Given in General Practice 1991–1999
By Dr Stephen Longworth MBChB MSc MRCGP DM-S Med DPCR FSOM

Region	Number of injections	%	
Shoulder	898	43	Upper limb 73%
Elbow	255	12	
Wrist/Hand	366	18	
Hip	103	5	Lower limb 27%
Knee	324	16	
Ankle/Foot	132	6	
Total	**2078**	**100**	

TOP SIX INJECTIONS

Chronic subdeltoid bursitis	546	(26% of Total peripheral injections)
Shoulder capsulitis	268	
Knee osteoarthritis (OA)	241	
Tennis elbow	186	
Trapezio metacarpal joint OA	103	
Plantar fasciitis	88	
Total	**1432**	**(69% of Total peripheral injections)**

APPENDIX 2

WEBSITES

The ILAR (International League of Associations for Rheumatology) 'Gateway to World Rheumatology' (www.ilar.org) is an excellent place to start, with comprehensive links to other sites and on-line journals.

OTHER SITES/ADDRESSES OF INTEREST

Annals of the Rheumatic Diseases	ard.bmjjournals.com
British Institute of Musculoskeletal Medicine	bimm.org.uk
British Medical Journal	bmj.com
Centre For Evidence Based Medicine	www.cebm.jr2.ox.ac.uk
Cochrane Library	www.cochranelibrary.com
Medline National Electronic Library for Health	www.nelh-pc.nhs.uk
National Health Service	www.nhs.uk
National Sports Medicine Institute of the UK	www.nsmi.org.uk
Oxford Internet Pain Site	www.jr2.ox.ac.uk/Bandolier/painres/painpag/index.html
Primary Care Rheumatology Society	www.pcrsociety.com
WorldOrtho (The World of Orthopaedics & Sports Medicine)	www.worldortho.com

APPENDIX 3

MEDICOLEGAL CONSIDERATIONS

INJECTION THERAPY BY HEALTH PROFESSIONALS OTHER THAN DOCTORS

In 1995 the Chartered Society of Physiotherapy (CSP) brought injection therapy into the remit of appropriately trained chartered physiotherapists in the UK. It is now commonly used both in hospital outpatient departments and community settings. The NHS Plan (2000) envisages the breaking down of professional barriers and the extension of prescribing rights to health professionals other than doctors[142].

The most recent advice from The Medical Defence Union (1999) is that a doctor delegating a task or referring a patient should ensure that the person to whom they are delegating or referring is competent[21] and is registered with a statutory regulatory body. Chartered physiotherapists working outside the NHS are personally liable for any claims arising out of their negligent acts or omissions and require personal indemnity, while those working within the NHS are indemnified by their employer.

GROUP PROTOCOLS

In the UK, recent changes to the Medicines Act (1968) allow doctors to sign group protocols. These allow other clinicians to administer medicines to groups of patients rather than named individuals. According to the Medicines Control Agency, to be lawful (from 9th August 2000), a group protocol should include:

- the signature of a doctor
- signature by an appropriate health organization
- the name of the business to which the direction applies
- the date the direction comes into force and the expiry date
- a description of the medicine to which the direction applies
- the clinical condition or situation to which the direction applies
- clinical criteria under which the patient is eligible for treatment
- exclusions from treatment under direction
- class of health professional who may supply or administer the medicine
- circumstances in which further advice should be sought from a doctor
- details of maximum dosage, quantity, pharmaceutical form and strength, route of administration, frequency and duration of administration
- relevant warnings
- details of any necessary follow-up action
- arrangements for referral for medical advice
- a statement for the records to be kept for audit arrangements.

REFERENCES

1. Anon. Articular and periarticular corticosteroid injection. *Drugs and Therapeutics Bulletin* 1995;33(9):67–70

2. Assendelft WJJ, Hay EM, Adshead R, Bouter LM. Corticosteroid injections for lateral epicondylitis: a systemic overview. *British Journal of General Practice* 1996;46:209–216

3. Van der Hijden GJMG, Van der Windt DAWM, Kleijnen J et al. Steroid injections for shoulder disorders: a systematic review of randomized clinical trials. *British Journal of General Practice* 1996;46:309–316

4. van der Windt DAWM, Koes BW, Deville W et al. Effectiveness of corticosteroid injections versus physiotherapy for treatment of painful stiff shoulder in primary care: randomised trial. *British Medical Journal* 1998;317:1292–1296

5. Dando P, Green S, Price J. *Problems in General Practice – Minor Surgery.* London; The Medical Defence Union 1997

6. Winters JC, Sobel JS, Groenier KH et al. Comparison of physiotherapy manipulation and corticosteroid injection for treating shoulder complaints in general practice: randomised single blind study. *British Medical Journal* 1997;314:1320–1325

7. Hay EM, Paterson SM, Lewis M et al. Pragmatic randomised controlled trial of local corticosteroid injection and naproxen for treatment of lateral epicondylitis of elbow in primary care. *British Medical Journal* 1999;319:964–968

8. Verhaar JAN, Walenkamp GHIM, van Mameren H et al. Local corticosteroid injection versus Cyriax type physiotherapy for tennis elbow. *Journal of Bone and Joint Surgery (Br)* 1995;77:128–132

9. Haslock I, Macfarlane D, Speed C. Intraarticular and soft tissue injections: a survey of current practice. *British Journal of Rheumatology* 1995;34:449–452

10. Marx RG, Bombardier C, Wright JG. What do we know about the reliability and validity of physical examination tests used to examine the upper extremity? *Journal of Hand Surgery* 1999;24A:185–193

11. Bamji AN, Erhardt CC, Price TR, Williams PL. The painful shoulder: can consultants agree? *British Journal of Rheumatology* 1996;35:1172–1174

12. Jones A, Regan M, Ledingham J et al. Importance of placement of intra-articular steroid injections. *British Medical Journal* 1995;307:1329–1330

13. Eustace JA, Brophy DP, Gibney RP et al. Comparison of the accuracy of steroid placement with clinical outcome in patients with shoulder symptoms. *Annals of the Rheumatic Diseases* 1997;56:59–63

14. Hollingworth GR, Ellis RM, Hattersley TS. Comparison of injection techniques for shoulder pain: results of a double blind randomised study. *British Medical Journal* 1983;287:1339–1341

15. Bliddal H. Placement of intra-articular injections verified by mini air-arthrography. *Annals of the Rheumatic Diseases* 1999;58:641–643

16. Kane D, Greaney T, Bresnihan B et al. Ultrasound guided injection of recalcitrant plantar fasciitis. *Annals of the Rheumatic Diseases* 1998;57:383–384

17. Winters JC, Jorritsma W, Groenier KH et al. Treatment of shoulder complaints in general practice: long term results of a randomised, single blind study comparing physiotherapy, manipulation, and corticosteroid injection. *British Medical Journal* 1999;318:1395–1396

18. Winters JC, Sobel JS, Groenier KH et al. The long term course of shoulder complaints: a prospective study in general practice. *Rheumatology* 1999;38:160–163

19. Bjorkenheim JM, Paavolainen P, Ahovuo J, Slatis P. Surgical repair of the rotator cuff and surrounding tissues. Factors influencing the results. *Clinical Orthopathology* 1988;236:148–153

20. Watson M. Major ruptures of the rotator cuff. The results of surgical repair in 89 patients. *Journal of Bone and Joint Surgery (Br)* 1985;67(4):618–624

21. ACPOM *A Clinical Guideline for the Use of Injection Therapy by Physiotherapists.* London; The Chartered Society of Physiotherapy 1999

22. Weale A, Bannister GC. Who should see orthopaedic outpatients – physiotherapists or surgeons? *Annals of the Royal College of Surgeons of England* 1994;77 (suppl):71–73

23. Dyce C, Biddle P, Hall K et al. Evaluation of extended role of physio and occupational therapists in rheumatology practice. *British Journal of Rheumatology* 1996 (April, suppl 1: abstracts):130

24. Hattam P, Smeatham An Evaluation of an orthopaedic screening service in primary care. *British Journal of Clinical Governance* 1999;4(2)45–49

25. Daker-White G, Carr AJ, Harvey I et al. A randomised controlled trial – shifting boundaries of doctors and physiotherapists in orthopaedic outpatient departments. *Journal of Epidemiology and Community Health* 1999;53:643–650

26. Haynes JC Jnr. Adrenocorticotrophic hormone; adrenocortical steroids and their synthetic analogues, inhibitors of the synthesis and actions of adrenocortical hormones. In: Godman AG et al (eds) *Godman and Gilman's Pharmacological Basis of Therapeutics,* 8th Edn. New York City; Pergamon Press 1990: pp 1431–1469

27. Coombes GM, Bax DE. The use and abuse of steroids in rheumatology. *Reports on the Rheumatic Diseases (Series 3). Practical Problems (No. 8)* 1996

28. Clarke A, Allard L, Braybrooks B. *Rehabilitation in Rheumatology – The Team Approach.* London; Martin Dunitz 1987: pp 147–153

29. Hollander JL, Brown EM, Jester RA et al. Hydrocortisone and cortisone injected into arthritic joints; comparative effects of a use of hydrocortisone as a local anti-arthritis agent. *Journal of the American Medical Association* 1951;147:1269

30. Kendall PH. Triamcinalone hexacetonide – a new cortico-steroid for intra-articular therapy. *American Physiology and Medicine* 1967;9:55–58

31. Gray RG, Gottlieb NL. Basic sscience and pathology: intra-articular corticosteroids, an updated assessment. *Clinical Orthopaedics and Related Research* 1982;177:235–263

32. Creamer P. Intra-articular corticosteroid injections in osteoarthritis: do they work, and if so, how? *Annals of the Rheumatic Diseases* 1997;56:634–636

33. Goulding NJ. Anti-inflammatory corticosteroids. *Reports on the Rheumatic Diseases (Series 3). Topical Reviews (No. 18)* 1999:1

34. Owen DS. Aspiration and injection of joints and soft tissues. In: Kelly WN et al (eds) *Textbook of Rheumatology,* 5th Edn. New York; WB Saunders 1997: pp 591–608

35. Simone J. The principles of corticosteroid injection therapy in musculoskeletal medicine. *Journal of Orthopaedic Medicine* 1993;15(3):56–58

36. *British National Formulary* No 40 (Sept 2000) p 463 BMA/RPSGB, London

37. Jones A, Doherty M. Intra-articular corticosteroid injections are effective in OA but there are no clinical predictors of response. *Annals of the Rheumatic Diseases* 1996;55:829–832

38. Hochberg MC, Altman RD, Brandt RD et al. Guidelines for the medical management of osteoarthritis. Part II osteoarthritis of the knee. *Arthritis and Rheumatism* 1995;38(11):1541–1546

39. Leadbetter W. Anti-inflammatory therapy in sports injury. *Clinics In Sports Medicine* 1995;14:(2)353–410

40. Kirwan JR, Rankin E. Intraarticular therapy in osteoarthritis. *Baillière's Clinical Rheumatology* 1997;11(4):769–794

41. Dorman T, Ravin T. *Diagnosis and Injection Techniques in Orthopaedic Medicine.* Baltimore, Maryland; Williams and Wilkins 1991: pp 33–34

42. Daley CT, Stanish WD. Soft tissue injuries: overuse syndromes. In: Bull RC (ed) *Handbook Of Sports Injuries.* New York; McGraw Hill 1998: p 185

43. Pelletier JP, Pelletier JM. Proteoglycan degrading metalloprotease activity in human osteoarthritis cartilage and the effect of intraarticular steroid injections. *Arthritis and Rheumatism* 1987;30(5):541–549

44. Jubb RW. Anti-rheumatic drugs and articular cartilage. *Reports on the Rheumatic Diseases (Series 2). Topical Reviews (No. 20)* 1992

45. Chard MD, Cawston TE, Riley GP et al. Rotator cuff degeneration and lateral epicondylitis: a comparative histological study. *Annals of the Rheumatic Diseases* 1994;53:30–34

46. Riley GP, Harrall RL, Constant CR et al. Tendon degeneration and chronic shoulder pain: changes in the collagen composition of the human rotator cuff tendons in rotator cuff tendinitis. *Annals of the Rheumatic Diseases* 1994;53:359–366

47. Riley GP, Harrall RL, Constant CR et al. Glycosaminoglycans of human rotator cuff tendons: changes with age and in chronic rotator cuff tendinitis. *Annals of the Rheumatic Diseases* 1994;53:367–376

48. Khan KM, Cook JL, Bonar F et al. Histopathology of common tendinopathies. *Sports Medicine* 1999;27(6):393–408

49. Khan KM, Cook JL, Maffulli N, Kannus P. Where is the pain coming from in tendinopathy? It may be biochemical, not structural in origin. *British Journal of Sports Medicine* 2000;34(2):81–83

50. Blyth T, Hunter JA, Stirling A. Pain relief in the rheumatoid knee after steroid injection: a single blind comparison of hydrocortisone succinate, and triamcinolone acetonide or hexacetonide. *British Journal of Rheumatology* 1994;33(5):461–463

51. Piotrowski M, Szczepanski I, Dmoszynska M. Treatment of rheumatic conditions with local instillation of betamethasone and methylprednisolone: comparison of efficacy and frequency of irritative pain reaction. *Rheumatologia* 1998;36:78–84

52. Birrer RB. Aspiration and corticosteroid injection. *Physiology and Sports Medicine* 1992;20(12):57–71

53. Barry M, Jenner JR. Pain in the neck, shoulder and arm (ABC of Rheumatology). *British Medical Journal* 1995;310:183–186

54. Mens JMA, De Wolf AN, Berkhout BJ, Stam HJ. Disturbance of the menstrual pattern after local injection with triamcinolone acetonide. *Annals of the Rheumatic Diseases* 1998;57:700

55. Drury PL, Howlett TA. Endocrinology. In: Kumar P, Clark M (eds) *Clinical Medicine,* 4th Edn. Edinburgh; W B Saunders 1998: p 941

56. Lazarevic MB, Skosey JL, Djordjevic-Denic G. Reduction of cortisol levels after single intra-articular and intramuscular steroid injection. *American Journal of Medicine* 1995;99(4):370–373

57. Pullar T. Routes of drug administration: intra-articular route. *Prescribers' Journal* 1998;38(2):123–126

58. Taylor HG, Fowler PD, David MJ, Dawes PT. Intra-articular steroids: confounder of clinical trials. *Clinical Rheumatology* 1991;10(1):38–42

59. Fisher M. Treatment of acute anaphylaxis. *British Medical Journal* 1995;311:731–733

60. Ewan PW. Anaphylaxis (ABC of allergies). *British Medical Journal* 1998;316:1442–1445

61. Vervloet D, Durham S. Adverse reactions to drugs (ABC of Allergies). *British Medical Journal* 1998;316:1511–1514

62. Wallace WA. (letter) *British Medical Journal* 2000;320 4th March

63. Binder AI, Hazleman BL. Lateral humeral epicondylitis – a study of natural history and the effect of conservative therapy. *British Journal of Rheumatology* 1983;22:73–76

64. Kumar N, Newman R. Complications of intra- and peri-articular steroid injections. *British Journal of General Practice* 1999;49:465–466

65. Newman RJ. Local skin depigmentation due to corticosteroid injections. *British Medical Journal* 1984;288:1725–17260

66. Price R, Sinclair H, Heinrich I, Gibson T. Local injection treatment of tennis elbow – hydrocortisone, triamcinolone and lignocaine compared. *British Journal of Rheumatology* 1991;30:39–44

67. Lanyon P, Regan M, Jones A, Doherty M. Inadvertent intra-articular injection of the wrong substance. *British Journal of Rheumatology* 1997;36:812–813

68. Gray RG, Tenenbaum J, Gottlieb NL. Local corticosteroid injection therapy in rheumatic disorders. *Seminars in Arthritis and Rheumatism* 1981;10:231–54

69. Cameron G. Steroid arthropathy: myth or reality? *Journal of Orthopaedic Medicine* 1995; 17(2):51–55

70. Gosal HS, Jackson AM, Bickerstaff DR. Intra-articular steroids after arthroscopy for osteoarthritis of the knee. *Journal of Bone and Joint Surgery (Br)* 1999;81:952–954

71. Currey HLF, Hull S. Management and referral. In: *Rheumatology for General Practitioners*. Oxford: 1987: p 223

72. Doherty M, Hazleman B, Hutton CW et al. Principles of joint aspiration and steroid injection. In: *Rheumatology Examination and Injection Techniques*. London; WB Saunders 1992: p 123–127

73. Cooper C, Kirwan JR. Risks of corticosteroid therapy. *Clinical Rheumatology* 1990;19:305–332

74. Smith AG, Kosygan K, Williams H, Newman RJ. Common extensor tendon rupture following corticosteroid injection for lateral tendinosis of the elbow. *British Journal of Sports Medicine* 1999;33:423–425

75. Shrier I, Gordon O. Achilles tendon: are corticosteroid injections useful or harmful? *Clinical Journal of Sports Medicine* 1996;6:245–250

76. Mahler F, Fritsch YD. Partial and complete ruptures of the Achilles tendon and local corticosteroid injections. *British Journal of Sports Medicine* 1992;26:7–14

77. Acevedo JI, Beskin JL. Complications of plantar fascia rupture associated with corticosteroid injection. *Foot and Ankle International* 1998;19:91–97

78. Fredberg U. Local corticosteroid injection in sport: review of literature and guidelines for treatment. *Scandinavian Journal of Medicine and Science in Sport* 1997;7:131–139

79. Cyriax JH, Cyriax PJ. Principles of treatment. In: *Illustrated Manual of Orthopaedic Medicine*. Butterworths 1983: p 22

80. Read MTF. Safe relief of rest pain that eases with activity in achillodynia by intrabursal or peritendinous steroid injection: the rupture rate was not increased by these steroid injections. *British Journal of Sports Medicine* 1999;33:134–135

81. Mottram DR (ed). *Drugs in Sport,* 2nd Edn. London: E & FN Spon 1996

82. Hughes RA. Septic arthritis. *Reports on the Rheumatic Diseases (Series 3). Practical Problems (No. 7)* 1996:1

83. Hollander JL. Intrasynovial corticosteroid therapy in arthritis. *Maryland State Medical Journal* 1970;19:62–70

84. Seror P, Pluvinage P, Lecoq F et al. Frequency of sepsis after local corticosteroid injection (an inquiry on 1,160,000 injections in rheumatological private practice in France). *Rheumatology* 1999;38:1272–1274

85. von Essen R, Savolainen HA. Bacterial infection following intra-articular injection. *Scandinavian Journal of Rheumatology* 1989;18:7–12

86. Case History 1: Inadequate asepsis? *Journal of the Medical Defence Union* 1995;11(1):11

87. Gardner GC, Weisman MH. Pyarthrosis in patient with rheumatoid arthritis; a report of 13 cases and a review of the literature from the past 40 years. *American Journal of Medicine* 1990;88:503–511

88. Knight DJ, Gilbert FJ, Hutchison JD. Lesson of the week: septic arthritis in osteoarthritic hips. *British Medical Journal* 1996;313:40–41

89. Ryan MJ, Kavanagh R, Wall PG, Hazleman BL. Bacterial joint infections in England and Wales: analysis of bacterial isolates over a four year period. *British Journal of Rheumatology* 1997;36:370–373

90. Tramer MR, Moore RA, Reynolds JM, McQuay HJ. Quantitative estimation of rare adverse events which follow a biological progression: a new model applied to chronic NSAID use. *Pain* 2000;85:169–182

91. *British National Formulary* No 40 (Sept 2000) p 582 BMA/RPSGB, London

92. Corrigan B, Maitland GD. Management. *Practical Orthopaedic Medicine.* Oxford; Butterworth Heinemann 1983: p 21

93. Kannus P, Jarvinen M, Niittymaki S. Long- or short-acting anesthetic with corticosteroid in local injections of overuse injuries? A prospective, randomized, double-blind study. *International Journal of Sports Medicine* 1990;11(5):397–400

94. Soluaborn S et al. Cortisone injection with anaesthetic additives for radial epicondylalgia. *Clinical Orthopaedics & Related Research* 1995;316:99–105

95. Jacobs LGH, Barton MAJ, Wallace WA et al. Intraarticular distension and steroids in the management of capsulitis of the shoulder. *British Medical Journal* 1991;302:1498–1501

96. Mulcahy KA, Baxter AD, Oni OOA, Finlay D. The value of shoulder distension arthrography with intra-articular injection of steroid and local anaesthetic: a follow-up study. *British Journal of Radiology* 1993;67:263–266

97. *British National Formulary* No 40. (Sept 2000) pp 454, 460, 464, 585 BMA/RPSGB, London

98. Watts RW, Silagy CA. A meta-analysis on the efficacy of epidural corticosteroids in the treatment of sciatica. *Anaesthesia and Intensive Care* 1995;23:564–569

99. McQuay HJ, Moore RA. Epidural steroids for sciatica. *Anaesthesia and Intensive Care* 1996;24:284–285 (letter)

100. Anon. Hyaluronan or hylans for knee osteoarthritis? *Drugs and Therapeutics Bulletin* 1999;37(9):71–72

101. Gado K, Emery P. Intra-articular guanethidine injection for resistant shoulder pain: a preliminary double blind study of a novel approach. *Annals of the Rheumatic Diseases* 1996;55:199–201

102. Heuft-Dorenbosch LLJ, deVet HCW, van der Linden S. Yttrium radiosynoviorthesis in the treatment of knee arthritis in rheumatoid arthritis: a systematic review. *Annals of the Rheumatic Diseases* 2000;59:583–586

103. Aronson JK. Where name and image meet – the argument for 'adrenaline'. *British Medical Journal* 2000; 320:506–509

104. Cawley PJ, Morris IM. A study to compare the efficacy of two methods of skin preparation prior to joint injection. *British Journal of Rheumatology* 1992;31:847–848

105. Dacre JE, Beeney N, Scott DL. Injections and physiotherapy for the painful stiff shoulder. *Annals of the Rheumatic Diseases* 1989;48:322–325

106. Smith RW et al. Methods of skin preparation prior to intra-articular injection. (letter) *British Journal of Rheumatology* 1993;32(7)648

107. Handwashing Liaison Group. Hand washing. *British Medical Journal* 1999;318:686

108. Hartley JC, Mackay AD, Scott GM Wrist watches must be removed before washing hands. (letter) *British Medical Journal* 1999;318:328

109. Golding DN. Local corticosteroid injections. *Reports on the Rheumatic Diseases (Series 2). Practical Problems* (No. 19) 1991:1

110. Liang MH, Sturock RD. Evaluation of musculoskeletal symptoms. In: Klippel JH, Dieppe PA (eds). *Practical Rheumatology.* London; Mosby 1995: p 11

111. Baker L. *ACPOM Journal* January 1999;7:42–48

112. Department of Health. *Immunisation Against Infectious Diseases,* 2nd Edn. London; HMSO 1994:pp 38–41

113. Ewan PW. Treatment of anaphylactic reactions. *Prescribers' Journal* 1997;37:(3):125–132

114. Sander JWAS, O'Donaghue MF. Epilepsy: getting the diagnosis right. *British Medical Journal* 1997;314:158–159

115. Snashall D. Occupational infections (ABC of work related disorders). *British Medical Journal* 1996;313:553

116. UK Departments of Health. *Guidance for Clinical Health Care Workers: Protection Against Infection with Blood-borne Viruses.* London: HMSO 1998 (Online. Available: http://www.open.gov.uk/doh/chcguid1.htm)

117. Easterbrook P, Ippolito G. Prophylaxis after occupational exposure to HIV. *British Medical Journal* 1997; 315:557–558

118. Faher H, Rentsch HV, Gerber NJ et al. Knee effusion and reflex inhibition of the knee joint. *Journal of Bone and Joint Surgery (Br)* 1988;70:635–637

119. Spencer J et al. Knee joint effusion and quadriceps reflex inhibition in man. *Archives of Physical and Medical Rehabilitation* 1984;65:171–177

120. Weitoft T, Uddenfeldt P. Importance of synovial fluid aspiration when injecting intra-articular corticosteroids. *Annals of the Rheumatic Diseases* 2000;59:233–235

121. Dieppe P, Swan A. Identification of crystals in synovial fluid. *Annals of the Rheumatic Diseases* 1999;58:261–263

122. Shmerling RH, Delbanco TL, Tosteson AN, Trentham DE. Synovial fluid tests – what should be ordered? *Journal of the American Medical Association* 1990;264:1009–1014

123. Von Essen R, Holtta A. Improved method of isolating bacteria from joint fluids by the use of blood culture bottles. *Annals of the Rheumatic Diseases* 1986;45:454–457

124. Stell IM, Gransden WR. Simple tests for septic bursitis: comparative study. *British Medical Journal* 1998; 316:1877

125. Varley GW, Needoff M, Davis TR, Clay NR. Conservative management of wrist ganglia: aspiration versus steroid infiltration. *Journal of Hand Surgery (Br)* 1997;22(5):636–637

126. Jones D, Chattopadhyay. Suprascapular nerve block for the treatment of frozen shoulder in primary care: a randomized trial. *British Journal of General Practice* 1999;49:39–41

127. Samanta A, Beardsley J. Sciatica: which intervention? *British Medical Journal* 1999;319:302–303

128. Bush K, Hillier S. A controlled study of caudal epidural injections of triamcinolone plus procaine for the management of intractable sciatica. *Spine* 1991;16(5):572–575

129. Koes B, Scholten RPM, Mens JMA, Bouter LM. Efficacy of epidural steroid injections for low back pain and sciatica: a systematic review of randomised clinical trials. *Pain* 1995;63:279–288

130. Carette S, Leclaire R, Marcoux S, et al. Epidural corticosteroid injections for sciatica due to herniated nucleus pulposus. *New England Journal of Medicine* 1997;336(23):1634–1640

131. Slosar PJ, White AH, Wetzel FT. Controversy – the use of selective nerve root blocks: diagnostic, therapeutic or placebo? *Spine* 1998;20:2253–2256

132. Riew KD, Yin Y, Gilula L et al. The effect of nerve root injections on the need for operative treatment of lumbar radicular pain. A prospective, randomised, controlled, double blind study. *Journal of Bone and Joint Surgery (Am)* 2000;82A:1589–1593

133. Nelemans PJ, de Bie RA, de Vet HCW, Sturmans F. Injection therapy for subacute and chronic benign low back pain (Cochrane Review). In: The Cochrane Library, Issue 4, 2000. Oxford: Update Software

134. Carette S, Marcoux S, Truchon R et al. A controlled trial of corticosteroid injections into facet joints for chronic low back pain. *New England Journal of Medicine* 1991;325(14):1002–1007

135. Ferner RE. Prescribing licensed medicines for unlicensed indications. *Prescribers' Journal* 36(2):73–78

136. Wildsmith JA. Routes of drug administration: 6. Intrathecal and epidural injection. *Prescribers' Journal* 36(2):110–115

137. Price CM, Rogers PD, Prosser ASJ, Arden NK. Comparison of the caudal and lumbar approaches to the epidural space. *Annals of the Rheumatic Diseases* 2000:879–882

138. Cyriax J. Epidural injection. In: *Textbook of Orthopaedic Medicine*, Vol 2, 11th Edn. London; Baillière Tindall 1984: p. 178

139. Bryan BM, Lutz C, Lutz GE. Fluoroscopic assessment of epidural contrast spread after caudal injection. *Journal of Orthopaedic Medicine* 2000;22(2):38–41

140. Dorman T, Ravin T. Treatment. In: *Diagnosis and Injection Techniques in Orthopaedic Medicine*. Baltimore, Maryland; Williams and Wilkins 1991: p. 34

141. Dechow E, Davies RK, Carr AJ, Thompson PW. A randomised, double blind, placebo controlled trial of sclerosing injections in patients with chronic low back pain. *Rheumatology* 1999;38:1255–1259

142. Department of Health. *The NHS Plan. A plan for investment. A plan for reform.* London:The Stationery Office; 2000

INDEX

Page numbers in italic print refer to tables and illustrations.